8/18/2000

To Ethel,
thank you for being
such good neighbors to
the Dormans!
Blessings
Shirley Jay Shaw

The Rakhma Story

The Rakhma Story

Unconditional Love and Caring
for People with Alzheimer's Disease and Dementia

by Shirley Joy Shaw
as told to Lynn Baskfield

1999
Galde Press, Inc.
Lakeville, Minnesota, U.S.A.

First Edition
First Printing, 1999

Grateful acknowledgment is made for permission to reprint from the following:
"Free to Be…A Family." Copyright © 1983 MS. Foundation for Women, Inc.
Used by permission.
"Self Portrait" by David Whyte. In *Fire in the Earth,* copyright © 1992 David
Whyte. Used by permission of Many Rivers Press.

Library of Congress Cataloging-in-Publication Data
Shaw, Shirley Joy
    The Rakhma story : unconditional love and caring for people with
Alzheimer's disease and dementia / by Shirley Joy Shaw as told to
Lynn Baskfield.
        p. cm.
    ISBN 1–880090–83–X (trade pbk.)
    1. Alzheimer's disease—Patients—Home care. 2. Alzheimer's
disease—Nursing. 3. Alzheimer's disease—Patients—Rehabilitation.
I. Baskfield, Lynn. II. Title.
RC523.S53   1998
362.1'96831—dc21   98–54693
                                                                           CIP

Galde Press, Inc.
PO Box 460
Lakeville, Minnesota 55044–0460

This book is dedicated to my grandmother, Alma D. Carlson.
The unconditional love, faith, and fun she
taught me has been the fabric of my life.
I hear her favorite Psalm, 121, as I go about my work.

I will lift up my eyes to the hills—from whence comes my help.
My help comes from the Lord, who made heaven and earth.
Verses 1 and 2

Contents

Acknowledgments

Shirley

My gratitude to the many people who helped in the beginning stages of Rakhma: Edith Stauffer, my inspiration who taught unconditional love; Dr. Schuller for his Sunday messages that encouraged me to "go for it!"; the many caregivers in my home care service, especially at the Littlejohn's home—Marie T., Marie A., Kathryn, Catherine, David, Jude, Thelma, and others. I appreciate the contributions of the many others who helped launch Rakhma Home I: Lynn Baskfield, Becky and Larry Dorman, Pam Boyce, Mary Dobbins, and Terry Johnson. I couldn't have done this without my first Board of Directors, Sherril Garahan, Jean Taylor, Mary Ondov, Chuck Smith, and Gloria Feik, and all the other dedicated board members throughout the years. Many thanks to my first volunteer, Barb Norling, and my volunteer business plan consultant Marybeth Hasse, and to my special cooks: my sisters Bettylou Freudenrich, Jean Taylor, and my mom Evelyn Hill. I am indebted to my supportive elders, Mabel Rhode and Stutsky Armstead for their wisdom and friendship. I also want to thank our many residents and their supportive family members.

Other important people during the growing pains of Rakhma were Dick Wiessner, Barbara Kellot, the Ramsey County licensing angel Cindy Brehm, our accounting angel Paul Tesserk and the Minnetonka State Bank, and the Minnesota Lakes Alzheimer's Association. Heartfelt thanks to many staff members, particularly Seini Taufeulungaki, June Webb Notermann, Nat Norris, Siri Hoffart, Judy Melinat, Shari Skally, and Elizabeth Manfredi, who were all so very important to the success of Rakhma throughout the years. There are so many special people that I can't begin to name them all, but I extend my sincerest gratitude to each and every one of you. As my elder friend Stutsky taught me, "What blesses one, blesses all."

I would like to acknowledge my four children, Cindy, Becky, Liz, and James, who have taught me many lessons in patience and love. I am very proud of each one of you. And those precious ones, my twelve grandchildren: Ben, Naomi, Seth, Laura, Ruth, David, Mandy, Luke, Zackary, Sammi Jo, Alexa Joy, and baby Mackenzie—what a joy they add to my life.

And my deepest gratitude to our many guardian angels.

Lynn

It has been a privilege to have Shirley Joy Shaw as a friend, inspiration, and co-conspirator all these years. She is truly a kindred spirit. I am blessed by the unwavering support of my husband Bill. I saw in his creative soul my own and began to write, teach, and tell stories again. I am grateful to my two children, Louise and Shannon, whom I love beyond measure and of whom I am very proud. As for my mother, Dorothy, who touched me with her generosity, her grace, and her unflagging love, I am deeply grateful for having recognized her incredible beauty before she died. I thank Scott Edelstein for his wisdom and good humor as he guided Shirley and me through contractual details of collaboration and publication. And many thanks to Phyllis Galde for her life of service; for listening to the still, small voice within that led her to publishing; and for her commitment to publishing quality books that make a difference.

Preface

Alzheimer's disease is a problem for American society now. Somewhere between three and four million Americans currently have the disease. But what we are seeing in 1998 is only a shadow of the dilemma that we will face in thirty or forty years. The number of individuals with Alzheimer's will effectively double by the year 2030. Who is going to care for our elders with Alzheimer's disease? We desperately need new approaches to caring for our cognitively impaired elderly. That is what this book by Lynn Baskfield and Shirley Shaw is about.

Long ago, in the nineteenth century, the proportion of elders in society was quite small compared to the rest of the population. Our society was less mobile and less urban then. That Victorian ideal of caring for Grandma or Grandpa at home was much more feasible than it is today. In our mind's eye, though, the nineteenth century ideal of keeping one's family member at home is the paragon.

But, alas, we live in a fast paced, high pressure society where both spouses are likely to work and their aging parents might live a thousand miles away. We've come to rely more on others to provide care for our parents and grandparents. I know that sounds like a pejorative comment on our society, but I am merely stating our reality.

The current system of nursing home placement doesn't work very well now, and, as the number of elders increases, it will work even less well. Our system of state regulated nursing homes has its share of dedicated workers and determined administrators. But anyone who has been in a nursing home knows how impersonal and institutional they feel. And if you have ever questioned the ways that things are done in a nursing home, you will run right into the well-meaning but cumbersome and often burdensome regulations and rules. You find nursing staff spending more time with required paperwork than with the residents. You find rules that don't apply to your family member but which must be adhered to lest a state surveyor give the facility a black mark.

Shirley Shaw had a vision for Rakhma that was truly bold. She determined to create a home-like environment for elders with dementia. Such a home would not feel like a state hospital. It would feel more like a private residence. In our era of heavy state regulation, enforced by the fact that state governments hold the purse strings for most individuals in need of twenty-four hour care, it was truly bold and audacious of Shirley to think that she could create something that was different. Bureaucrats paid lip service to methods of care that were innovative, but they couldn't really allow innovative programs to exist if there was no government oversight. And if there was to be oversight, there would be regulations and restrictions and paperwork and extra costs and on and on, until the innovative program was either no different from a typical nursing home, or was out of business because it was too costly. Now, in the defense of bureaucrats, they are simply responding to their bosses—federal regulations, legislators, and the public—who want everything safe, even if it is costly and cumbersome and burdensome. But, despite all this, Shirley has succeeded in developing a series of homes for elderly demented individuals.

I am a physician who takes care of Alzheimer patients, and I have a feeling of deep frustration when faced with patients who need twenty-four hour care that the family can no longer provide. I really want to give families all of the resources that I have available to allow them to keep their family member at home. I know that in most of the families that I care for, not giving up is a major commitment. But I also know how hard it is for families as Alzheimer's disease moves into its severe stages. It can be so emotionally exhausting and physically draining that it is also my responsibility as a physician to say to a care-giving spouse, son or daughter, "Enough!" With the option of placement at a Rakhma home or similar type facility spawned by Shirley Shaw's success, I feel much better about the decisions to give up home care.

I salute Shirley Shaw and Lynn Baskfield and commend this book to readers who want to learn about a better way of caring for Alzheimer's disease and dementia.

—DAVID S. KNOPMAN, M.D.

Professor, Department of Neurology, University of Minnesota
Alzheimer's Disease Center

Foreword

Our society is aging. The social and economic consequences of this have yet to be fully appreciated. However, the increasing demands this places upon our health care system have already been felt for some time. When the oldest members of our society were born, it was typical for extended families to live together, often under the same roof. In large families, older brothers and sisters looked after their younger siblings, while adult children with families of their own were caregivers for elderly or infirm family members as well.

During the past century, however, the tradition of care in the home has been eroded as much by changes in demographics and societal values as by economic forces. In general, families have become smaller, and our society has become more mobile. Two-income families are no longer the exception, but rather a requirement to make ends meet. These and other factors have led over the past two generations to a shift of care delivery from home to institutional settings. Meanwhile, the institutions themselves have changed.

Most nursing homes in existence today were built to look and operate much like hospitals. Their original purpose was to house cognitively intact individuals recovering from medical illness. Because of society's collective inability or unwillingness to provide for our old and frail family members at home, nursing facilities became custodial housing sites for over one million elderly Americans, most suffering from Alzheimer's disease and related conditions. The unsuitability of this environment for many of the residents led inevitably to the increased use of physical and pharmacological restraints to control behavior, until strict federal standards were eventually enacted.

Nursing home care is expensive. The average person cannot afford to pay in excess of thirty thousand dollars per year to live in one. When the individual resident becomes impoverished, lacking any reasonable housing alternative, federal and state governments (through Medicaid) usually end up picking up the tab.

Hospital care is even more expensive, however. Amid a national clamor to curtail escalating health care costs, there has been a concerted shift in the provision of acute medical care away from hospitals and toward less expensive sites such as nursing homes. Consequently, the frail elderly, that segment of our society that was displaced a generation ago from their families and homes, is being displaced again, this time from the nursing home.

Within this context, *The Rakhma Story* is a chronicle of the future foretold. It is a story about the very best of human aspirations and hopes, about the building of a community: a community of kindness, compassion, and devotion. In essence, the community of man.

The people of Rakhma have created a social model of care that is fundamentally different from the traditional American medical model. Central to this new model is the importance of home. For an individual suffering from Alzheimer's disease or a similar condition, it is impossible to separate one's illness from one's environment. The provision of appropriate medical care can only occur in this context. Therefore, in an effort to insure the vitality of one's home regardless of the barriers imposed by cognitive impairment, the people of Rakhma have not only created a new home, they have reinvented the meaning of it. In so doing, they have enabled many to once again live private, dignified, and hopeful lives. At the same time, they have challenged the rest of us to re-examine the way we ourselves live.

As a geriatrician, it is my belief that no patients are more deserving of high quality, compassionate care, and none more grateful, than our elders and their families. I am excited and proud to be involved in the care of older patients. I relish the stories that each of us has to share. *The Rakhma Story* is worth the telling.

JONATHAN M. EVANS, M.D.
Geriatrician, Mayo Clinic, Rochester, Minnesota
Department of Internal Community Medicine

Introduction

For truly I tell you, if you have faith the size of a mustard seed you will say to this mountain, "Move from here to there," and it will move; and nothing will be impossible for you.

—Matthew 17:20

My grandmother lived in a cabin she helped build on the edge of Birch Lake in northern Minnesota. I remember the summers I spent with her. It seemed normal to me that an older woman would do what she did—chop wood for her stove, carry big buckets of water in from the lake in winter, take long walks in the woods, sit in a rocker reading her Bible, save her money in an old sock and count it every spring, saying, "I wonder how far this will take us." Grandma taught me that you can travel far on very little money and that nothing is impossible. Most importantly, through her unwavering faith and embracing presence in my life she taught me the meaning of unconditional love. A day never went by without her saying, "My goodness, I have so many blessings. There is so much to be grateful for!"

By the time I was fifteen, I had the woods and rocks and water in my soul. On my ambles through Grandma's woods, I remember being aware of walking softly underneath the trees, stepping gently over the moss and the deadwood, and watching the little wild critters scurry about. There was a hushed reverence that took my breath away, almost like being in a cathedral. I wrote an essay for school about how the woods gave me such peace. I had a desire to see the kind of peace and harmony I experienced in those woods manifested in the world around me. I got an A+ on my paper.

Albert Schweitzer was my hero. I read everything about him I could get my hands on. He had such talent. Not only was he was an accomplished organist, but he later became a theologian and philosopher. His reverence for life was an inspiration. He felt a further calling to help people in Africa, so he became a doctor. I wanted to do something meaningful, too, but I didn't know how at seventeen.

I thought, like a lot of other young women of my generation, that marrying, having children, and being a wife and mother was the only path open to me. I daydreamed about marrying a doctor or minister, which then would allow me to stand at the side of someone doing great work. I couldn't imagine that I could do something great by myself. Still, as I raised my four children, I sensed there was something more I was supposed to be doing.

I did a lot of volunteer work. When our family moved to Paris, I volunteered at the American School of Paris where my children were enrolled. When my children and I and two dogs returned to Minneapolis, I continued doing volunteer work. I volunteered at a local counseling service for youth and families. I drove senior citizens to doctors' appointments and to the grocery store. I answered phones on a crisis hot line. I spent many hours at a fine rehabilitation center aiding handicapped people in their exercise classes and assisting elderly people in the swimming pool.

At one agency where I volunteered extensively, I was aware of payday. At that time I was being supported by my former husband. I had a flash that if I went back to school, I could earn a salary, too. I saved for tuition out of my grocery money and enrolled in college.

It was winter quarter, one of those cold winters with lots of snow. The heater in my car didn't work. I drove from the suburb where I lived to classes in Minneapolis bundled in layers of clothing, sorrel boots, long underwear, and mittens. I'd pray a lot driving back and forth, worried that my car might break down.

It was also a time of healing from a broken marriage and getting to know my needs better. At home there were the four children and a menagerie of critters—dogs, cats, a boa constrictor, white mice, and guinea pigs. I remember thinking that raising four children was a challenge and that if I died tomorrow, what I did with my life was enough. I already was great. Aren't we all?

The first couple of years in college I trained to become a chemical dependency specialist. I took some women's studies. I also went to Outward Bound School, an outdoor skills training setting which helped give me the courage and confidence I needed to face challenges. It was there I made a new friend, Kitty Smith, who not only opened the door to twenty years of canoeing trips with a group of beautiful women, but who encouraged me as my vision of caring for people with memory loss became real.

Between leading youth groups at junior high schools and having four teenagers at home at the same time, life was intense. I didn't think I wanted the intensity of being a chemical dependency counselor, but what *did* I want to do for a career? Grandma's cabin was a healing place to make decisions. A trip there gave me new direction.

During that time I spent by the lake, sitting in the quiet, I remembered my volunteer work with the elderly and how much I loved it. I asked soul-searching questions. Can I have a career doing something I love doing? Can working with the elderly be a career for me? I didn't want to do elder care just because I was familiar with caregiving or because it felt comfortable. I wanted to be of service.

I concluded that I did want a career working with the elderly. They are a special group of people. I could be a voice for their dignity. I could be an advocate for their needs. Many of them have spent a lifetime caring for other people. I could give them the care they've given all these years. I could also give them lots of love. That was my decision.

I believe Rakhma was the work waiting to be done by me. I heard and responded. The time was right. Rakhma was not created by me. I was only an instrument to give care and to teach love. To follow this path has been a privilege. It took many dedicated people, prayers, and God's grace to do this work. I am eternally grateful for the opportunity to bring forth the Rakhma model. It is God's love expressed.

The journey continues to be a joy.

Blessings.

—SHIRLEY JOY SHAW

Chapter I

Beginnings

Tell Me Again About the House

Some hae meat
  and cannot eat
and some hae nae
  that wannet.

But we hae meat
  and we can eat,
so let the Lord
  be thanket.

—Scottish Table Grace

Rakhma began as a home-care "service with a heart," as my business card read. The card folded out to list all the help Rakhma could provide between 9:00 A.M. and 6:00 P.M. Lena and Douglas Littlejohn were the first total care case the fledgling service took on. My helpers and I began by dividing our time between meal preparation, showers and grooming, housecleaning and activities to provide mental and physical stimulation. I soon found that helping Lena and Doug required more hours, that the ebb and flow of their lives didn't compartmentalize into meal prep/grooming/cleaning. To respond to individual needs as they came and went meant honoring them as unique beings, and taking the time to really pay attention to them.

Doug Littlejohn was born in New Deer, Aberdeenshire, Scotland in 1889. Lena was of German descent, born and raised in Niagara Falls, Ontario. At age twenty, Doug left Scotland for the Niagara Falls area. He met Lena when they both landed parts in a musical play about gypsies. They fell in love and married in 1919.

On the advice of Doug's cousin Frank, they moved to Minneapolis in the mid-1920s—you could get work there, he said. Even though Doug had a job at a Canadian bank, times were getting harder. He went to work for the Federal Reserve Bank in Minneapolis as a self-titled accountant-book-keeper; then, during the 1930s, he kept accounts for the Red and White food stores. After that, he freelanced for a number of companies.

Lena worked part-time to help keep food on the table, selling San Moreno food products door to door until she worked up a steady clientele that placed their orders directly with her. She was a devoted homemaker with a strict routine: wash on Monday, iron on Thursday. She and Doug had three children between 1921 and 1926—June, Bill, and Jim.

Doug and Lena rented their homes until the mid-1940s. Even though things were tough financially, Lena made sure that the family always lived in a "nice" part of Minneapolis. When they bought their first home, they were as excited as a new bride and groom. Doug continued to work long hours, and Lena got a job at Powers Dry Goods Store, then Dayton's Department Store selling ladies better coats and suits.

Lena was raised in the Anglican church. However, Judson Memorial Community Church was within walking distance of their red brick home on 39th and Grand. She and Doug joined Judson because they didn't have a car to drive the distance to an Anglican church. She was hesitant at first, but since Judson was a *community* church she felt it would be acceptable. The Littlejohns developed a long and fruitful relationship with Judson Church that lasted until they died. Doug became a deacon. Lena sang in the choir.

Lena loved music. She had a trained contralto voice that became known throughout the city. She sang in the St. Paul Episcopal Boys Choir Adult Quartet and in the double quartet at Hennepin Avenue Methodist Episcopal Church. Both were paid positions that brought in money during the Depression. An unrelenting case of stage fright kept her from ever singing solo.

In her spare time, Lena enjoyed sewing. One of her daughter June's favorite memories is of a little coat and hat she crafted at Christmas for June's most loved doll.

Although both Lena and Doug worked very hard, there were vacations in rented cottages at nearby lakes. While Lena and Doug worked during the day in the city, the children, who were by then old enough to look after themselves, would sleep and play, then rush around cleaning up minutes before they knew their parents were to arrive at the end of the day. June remembers fishing sometimes with her dad on the lake and savoring the fish for supper that same night.

After Doug retired he became an avid gardener, getting down on his hands and knees, feeling the soil and lovingly breaking the clumps with his hands. When the children had all moved on, he grew a large and lovely garden behind the house. Lena tended the house plants. African violets and gloxinias, varieties some people have trouble growing, were among her favorites. She left the outdoor work to Doug, but often remarked on the beauty of "our" garden.

By the time I began working with the Littlejohns, they had sold their home and moved into an apartment that was smaller and easier to maintain. On my first visit, I found a tired, pale Doug and a depressed-looking Lena in a lot of pain. Meals on Wheels was their main sustenance, each eating half an entree at lunch and sometimes eating the other half for dinner. They sat together most of the day quietly passing the time.

Kathryn, one of the home-care team that worked with Doug and Lena, designed exercises especially for them, picking up on events from their lives. She used threshing movements that reminded them of the farms they grew up on, Scottish music that they loved, mental imagery that celebrated Doug's Scottish heritage and Lena's passion for beauty.

Thelma, the registered nurse who helped with care and assessment, observed that my service had a pattern of involvement that enhanced Lena and Doug's lives. They were happier than they had been in a long time; Lena would laugh and sing, and both seemed to look forward to the next day.

Doug was legally blind. Most afternoons, David Cheny, one of the helpers, took him to the pool in his apartment building to swim. Doug liked David, the company of another man, and he loved getting in the water. Coincidentally, David's parents had been members of the same church that Lena and Doug belonged to. He could talk about common experiences with Doug and share some memories. They became friends. Doug let David help him shower after their swim, trim his mustache, and do personal grooming tasks he wasn't as willing to let a woman helper do. Lena never went in the pool herself but she would go down and joke with the men from the vantage point of a deck chair.

From their ground-level apartment the Littlejohns could see Minnehaha creek winding its way east. Now, with their helpers, they were able to get outdoors. They could sit out on their patio, watch the ducks swim in the creek, and throw bread to them, one of Lena's favorite pastimes. Their conversations now lauded the beauty of the trees and flowers, the marvelous changing seasons. They went out on that patio until the weather turned cold enough to wear wool scarves and mittens. A world they had left behind reopened.

Doug had the frailer health. When he went into the hospital for a blood transfusion, I brought Lena over for a visit. "I want a big kiss," Lena coaxed as she plunked herself down on Doug's lap. The two of them brought smiles to the hospital aids and to my helpers. To watch two people in their nineties be so affectionate was a joy. One aid commented, "Those two just made my day."

There was a point when I became aware of what a difference my helpers and I were making in the Littlejohns' lives. As a helper sat at the kitchen table making up the grocery list, Lena might say, "I'm craving rutabagas." The helpers would see to it that she and Doug always had things from the store they wanted and meals that they liked. Even when they didn't feel like eating, they had at least chosen part of the meal.

They had days when they weren't in the best of spirits, but with my service helping them they became involved again in their lives. There was a

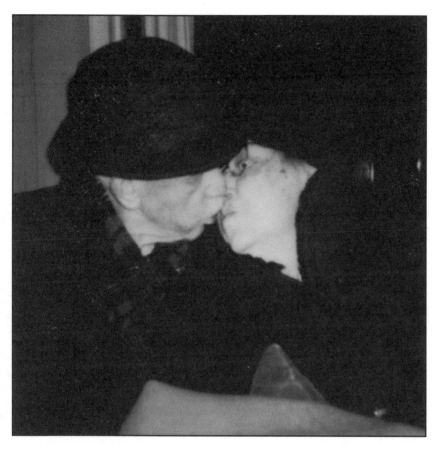

Doug and Lena Littlejohn sharing a kiss

lot of kidding around. My helpers and I would sit with them and invite them to tell their life stories on tape, capturing details of memorable dances and parties, their courtship and marriage, the joys and the setbacks of their years together. It was a source of joy to me that my helpers were all doing such a loving job in caring for them. Lena and Doug's family was pleased too.

Eventually I moved into doing twenty-four-hour care for the Littlejohns. Until then, I had not provided night care. Doug was falling more than before when he got up to use the bathroom. Lena often had chronic intestinal pain at night. Once into twenty-four-hour care, I had a better idea of the pattern of their lives. There was a lot of wakefulness at night. Doug's dreams had become so real to him that he often got up to open the front door for visitors who were not there. The last month before he and Lena moved into a nursing home Doug was having vivid dreams of a party and bagpipes playing. He talked about what Lena was wearing and all the people who where there, relatives and friends who had died a long time ago.

During one night shift I fell asleep on the floor. Through the heaviness of sleep I could hear music far away, but insistent. In a state between sleep and wakefulness, I lay there and listened to the music. The wail of bagpipes droned in the distance. In the waking state, the bagpipes disappeared and I couldn't hear them anymore. I wondered if, in that semi-sleeping state, I wasn't picking up bagpipes from Doug's dream. That's how it felt to me.

Helpers would talk about how Doug could see clouds and people that no one else saw. "Don't you see these people? They're all up there," he'd say, looking up at the ceiling.

"That's wonderful... I wish I could," Kathryn would reply, giving comfort and encouragement for the experience he was having.

A Celebration of Life

A week before Lena and Doug moved to a nursing home, my helpers and I hosted two celebrations of their life. Family members came. Staff members, a woman who is now a Rakhma board member, a neighbor, and some church friends came, too. The musical group, Aurora, brought harp, guitar, and autoharp and played in the living room. Singing and dancing was the order of the day, in honor of the parties, singing and dancing that over the years had always been an important part of Lena and Doug's life together. She still had that beautiful contralto voice that had once been known around the Twin Cities. A purple heather plant adorned the table, the best china was set out, and I made Scottish trifle, one of Lena and Doug's favorite desserts.

Jude, one of the home-care helpers, read a poem she had written in honor of Lena and Doug:

The great river of time has carried you
from those first waters where all is safe and warm
through many years and journeys,
through light and darkness, joy and suffering
through knowing and not knowing
the mysteries and secrets of yourselves
to this moment in the story of your lives
where you have come to full flowering.
You shall soon know again
the deep warm waters that wash and soothe
and surround the very heart of life;
where God is and home,
where you shall live in peace and light
more fully than any of us can imagine.
May your passing be as gentle as a sigh,
as soft as a breeze,
as clear as lake waters,
as safe as a loving embrace.
We will always know you are near.

"Oh, that is lovely, lovely," said Lena, when Jude was done. Then she read the poem herself, faltering at first as she groped for the words and the meaning, but soon hit her stride in her rich dramatic voice. A hush fell over the room.

The poem, the reminiscences, the clatter of dinner plates, and the little side conversations were all captured on tape that day. After Doug had gone to bed, home-care helper Kathryn and Lena got to talking about chicken.

"You ate chicken in bed once, remember?" Kathryn asked.

"Yes, I may have had it twice for all I know."

"You were telling me you were going to die that night and you told me all of the people for me to say good-bye to. But you still told me you wanted your fried chicken, so I brought it in and you ate it in bed."

"I remember that."

"We decided you probably weren't ready to die," interjected Marie, another helper. "It's the chicken that keeps you going."

With Lena there were silences in the conversation. She liked to chew on things, think them over a little. Everyone sat quietly while she did this.

"The old rooster," Lena asserted suddenly, referring to Doug. "It's not the chicken, it's that darn old rooster!" She slapped her knee and a hoot of laughter came out of her that shook the chandelier. She surprised herself and everyone else. The room roared, belly laughter out of control, subsiding a bit, then rising again.

"Oh, my, yes. That darn old rooster."

Doug died May 22, 1983, four weeks after going into the nursing home. After three and a half more months passed, Lena joined him in death. The Littlejohns' children felt their parents would have lived longer in the kind of group home I began to envision as Lena and Doug needed more and more care. They needed a small home that was full of life and love. The family would have liked them to be in a house like that, but I didn't find the right place in time. Rakhma Home 1 was formally dedicated to them when it opened December 1, 1984, and their memory lives in the bustle of the innovative setting they inspired.

Finding the House

For three years I looked for a house to buy, a home for the elderly. Realtors wanted twenty-five to thirty thousand dollars down on almost everything I thought would work, and I didn't have that kind of money. One day I saw a sign on a stately stucco and brick home on the corner of 43rd and Lyndale South that said "Easy Terms." That drew me in. I had admired the house before, just walking by, but that day I went up to the door and knocked. The

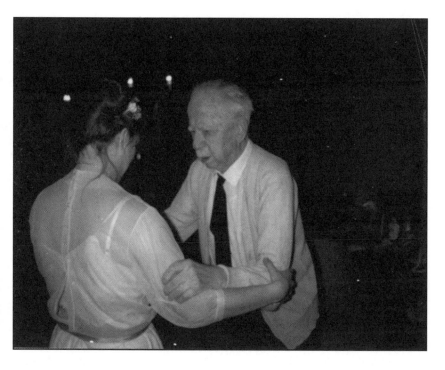

Kathryn Aronsen and Doug Littlejohn dancing at the Celebration of Life

house was vacant, but the owner happened to be there doing some painting. I stepped inside and knew it was the right house. I could turn the little library and the sun porch into first-floor bedrooms. There were two baths,
beautiful wood, lots of light, four bedrooms upstairs. It was not too big, not
too small. It was the first step to bringing my dream into reality.

I didn't have glasses then, although I needed them, and I thought the
Easy Terms sign read two thousand dollars instead of four thousand dollars
down. By then I had been through the house and fallen so in love with it that
Mr. Helgeson, the owner, realized I really wanted it. I didn't want to quib-
ble with the $106,000 asking price, but I didn't have four thousand dollars.
I thought I could come up with two thousand. He said, "I think I can do it
for two thousand dollars with an additional two thousand in nine months."

I went to my bank and tried to get a personal loan for two thousand dollars. They wanted me to sign my life away and put up my house, which I co-owned with Lynn Baskfield, for equity. I thought that was ridiculous. I had a little money in the bank from my home-care service, so I went to the other branch of the bank and found I had enough to make out a money order for two thousand dollars. Mr. Helgeson came over that night and I signed a purchase agreement. That day I bought a house on a contract for deed. Two thousand dollars down. The balance of the mortgage was due to balloon in a year and a half. (We'll talk about the implications of that later in chapter 4.)

Mr. Helgeson said that he didn't know what struck him. He had other offers after I had been to see the house, one from a lawyer who offered him more money. He really liked my attitude, though. He liked the idea that this would be a special place for the elderly, and that it would give people an alternative to a nursing home. "This is the most peaceful I've been in a long time," he said.

"I don't know why I'm doing this,' he said. He was trying hard to be not just a kind man, but a good businessman, and it seemed he couldn't be both at the same time.

Maybe he didn't know, but I knew. Our guardian angels have been with us since the beginning.

Having that first home was like having a first baby. You have theories about raising a child, perhaps even some baby-sitting experience, but you find out quickly that full time, day-to-day, hands-on responsibility is quite different from all your good ideas. Each day I learned that something else, something unexpected, was needed.

Even though Doug and Lena did not live to enjoy that first Rakhma home, Elan did. Elan was a delightful eighty-nine-year-old Swedish woman for whom I had provided home care.

Although Elan could never talk about her own difficulties, I noticed that her whole posture would change after someone spent time helping her in her apartment. Color came into her cheeks. She would become animated. My time as a care provider was officially over before noon, but I understood it was important for Elan to put her little cotton tablecloth on the table and share lunch with someone. So I stayed for lunches consisting of a boiled egg, cardamom bread with processed cheese, and good coffee. Elan, I saw, could be in charge at that time. Serving a lunch was something she was used to doing as a minister's wife. In her musical Swedish accent, Elan would talk of the past.

She was born and raised in Sweden. Her mother died when she was a child. As the oldest daughter in the family, she helped raise her nine brothers and sisters. When she was in her thirties, Elan met her future husband, a widowed minister, father of two children, pastor of a northern Minnesota church who was visiting relatives in Sweden. He showed an interest in her which, due to her shyness, she found flattering but awkward to return. As he was about to leave her village on the train, Elan momentarily forgot her shyness and raced across the field with a brilliant bouquet of wildflowers she had picked for him. Through the coach window she breathlessly offered her gift. Many letters made their way between Minnesota and Sweden after that: their courtship by mail culminated in a marriage proposal. Elan sailed for the states, and with her sweet minister, added seven children to his ready-made family of two.

Through our lunchtime talks, I saw what a hard worker Elan had always been and what a giving, loving spirit she had. Her door was always open to strangers and anyone who had any needs. Elan told stories of how, during the Depression, she would put out food for people who didn't have any from the big gardens she tended with her children.

At the time I met Elan, she lived in a high-rise apartment. Though there were activities for seniors she was not particularly interested in them. She would occasionally attend Bible study or prayer service, but it was a long walk down the hallway to get to the activity area. With chronic pain in her leg, she couldn't go the distance without discomfort. Pain at night was a constant companion.

It became apparent to me that Elan was lonely. She spoke with pride of her children and grandchildren. However, that wasn't enough to keep her from feeling displaced in her apartment building. She would never speak any ill will, but she missed people coming by to visit and the stimulation of an active household. Through Elan, I became more aware of the chronic loneliness and isolation that so many elderly people experience.

One day, in the midst of our luncheon conversation, I suddenly looked at Elan and said, "What would you think about living with other people in a house?" It was one of those moments of inspiration, of verbalizing the idea that had been niggling at me since caring for the Littlejohns.

It all just came out. I elaborated more about the house, that there would be people to talk to and eat with. We could cook our meals together, have some fun together, sing and read together. No one would have to be alone anymore.

"I don't even dare think about it," whispered Elan. She couldn't envision that it would ever happen for her.

Each time I came for lunch, the very last thing Elan would say before I left was, "Tell me again about the house."

At that point, I started looking for a house. It took three years to find one.

Clearly, alternatives were needed to the two living options currently available: staying at home or going into a nursing home. A small group home where people could care and share seemed a natural next step to the in-home services I had already been providing. Although I didn't find Rakhma Home 1 on Lyndale Avenue for three more years, those conversations with Elan began the search. Each time Elan, in her musical Swedish accent, asked, "Tell me again about the house," I would describe a home with wood floors and lace curtains, soup on the stove and a big dining room table to eat it on, flowers in the garden, music and laughter and more than enough love for everyone. Each telling honed the vision. It would be like a big, bustling family.

What Doug and Lena inspired, Elan confirmed—when people can no longer live at home, a home-like setting with twenty-four-hour care would be a good place to be. The next three years found Elan leaving the state to be with family; then, as her care needs increased, returning to Minnesota to be in a nursing home. After I bought Rakhma Home, the first of three community shared homes I have so far brought into being, I tracked Elan down through family members and asked if they would like her to live at "The House" for which she had been the inspiration.

Of course. Of course. There was no place Elan wanted to be more.

CHAPTER 2

Morning Always Comes
Rakhma, Inc.: The First Six Months

I have been on duty a lot and need to do some things for myself besides getting home. But whenever I share that with my special helper friends, I feel better. I feel they understand. Yet I know I will survive and the house will be filled and our financial situation will get better and better. I guess I've always been fairly optimistic. Maybe some people might say I've been naively optimistic at times.

—Shirley Shaw, Rakhma log book, April 1985

I was so new at this job and I couldn't always figure out what was going on. It was such a relief when the morning came, and it always did come. Now I can handle anything. Through this work I have become a totally different person.

—Seini Taufeulungaki,
House Manager, Rakhma Peace Home

Once I had a house, I felt like a Chinese plate spinner, keeping heavy pottery platters whirling at high speed on top of skinny little poles, running back and forth in response to the ones that were about to fall and at the same time remaining completely focused so that everything stayed in the air. Not only did I have to find residents, but I also had to recruit staff and furnish the house from top to bottom.

As for staff, I looked at the different helpers on my home-care team and saw that Seini Taufeulungaki was the person I wanted to work with me in the new home. Seini was a philosophical sort with an easygoing and positive attitude. Being from the South Pacific island of Tonga, she always brought to her work a deeply rooted tradition of respect and love for elders. I had a good rapport with Seini; we worked well together. Seini could be trusted not only with giving excellent care but also with holding the larger vision of what is possible for people when, no matter what their age or circumstance, they are treated with dignity and love. When I asked her to do this with me I remember her saying it would be an absolute pleasure and an honor. She started off with a salary of only six hundred dollars a month alternating care in the home with me. She would work so many days, twenty-four hours a day, and then I would work so many days, twenty-four hours. It was a lot of information gathering in the beginning. I was there when I wasn't working, too. It felt very good. We both were feeling very good about ourselves.

Rakhma Home I opened December 1, 1984. There were two residents, Elan and Hilda, another of my home-care clients. Hilda brought all the furniture from her apartment to Rakhma. Now there were a couch and chairs, rugs, tables, lamps, silverware, dishes, everything. It was wonderful. Not only did Rakhma have furniture, but Hilda felt very much at home with her things around her, and Elan did too. Everything was a bit broken in—comfortable, you might say. The things that were missing such as curtains and extra bedspreads, pan scrapers, and dishcloths, I bought with my trusty plastic card. The house quickly became a lovely place to live.

Having two residents was quite amazing. We were learning that it truly was twenty-four-hour care. The two ladies would be awake at different times, and Hilda would dress during the night. She was always trying to go somewhere, and she was so quiet about it. And Elan would dream and have pain in her legs. She would hobble up out of bed several times a night.

Seini's Adventure

"I was very young at the time," Seini relates, "so opening the house was like a new adventure. I felt like we were exploring a new frontier and we didn't have a map. When I look back, I see we didn't even know where we were

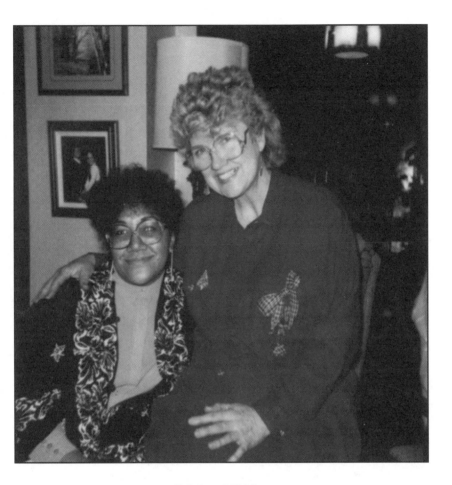

Seini and Shirley

going. On top of that, I was naive. Learning about the elderly with dementia was a whole new ball game, but I think I was good at it because I would always remember my parents and grandparents when I cared for the residents. It was a very simple philosophy, but it worked because I knew that Shirley wanted a family feeling and a home-like atmosphere. I didn't have to try too hard. I was just with the residents like I would be with my own family.

"I wrote a lot of funny notes because I was so new at it. The first day we were open I wrote:

"Dec. 1, 1984. Arrived shortly before noon. The ladies were expected to arrive before 1:00. Elan came first, then Hilda. All went well. It was fun having the family members puttering around the house, putting up last minute touches like pictures on the walls. The ladies, as I expected, were happy to be here, but at the same time, they had confusion, not knowing where they were. Anxiety. Will they like it here? Will they have regrets? Would they rather be where they were before? All in all it was a great day. I don't understand the dementia part, but we will make it somehow.

"I remember Elan waking up with that chronic pain in her leg and how she would want to get up at night. In March of '85 I wrote:

"Elan woke up twice wanting to talk about groceries and water.

"She was so busy at night. It was really challenging at first. One night, every fifteen minutes she was yelling out, 'Nurse, Nurse!' I thought I was going to go crazy. After a while she got out of bed, hobbled into the dining room, and did one big, loose BM in the middle of the floor. It was all so new to me I thought, 'What is going on?' In the middle of this I remember peeking out the dining-room window. It was spring outside. The trees were budding and I thought, 'My God, what beauty!' and here is this pile of shit at my feet and the house is just reeking. The saving grace for me was being able to appreciate the beauty, so I was able to come back, laugh at what happened, and be with Elan again. Such an innocent lady with a beautiful accent.

"It's mostly Elan I think of those first days because she was more demanding than Hilda. She would take over because she needed more. Hilda was more mellow. She would get up at night and dress for church, but we would tell her it wasn't time and she would go back to bed so as not to disturb anyone. I did home care for her before she came to Rakhma. We had a special bond. She would only let me do things for her, not anyone else.

"Hilda would say the same things over and over. 'Isn't it a beautiful day? Isn't that a beautiful sky?' She made the best dinner salads. She would stand in the kitchen and hum, shredding lettuce and tossing vegetables. Sometimes she would just hold my hand and hum. I could take her out for walks at thirty below and she wouldn't complain. She was a strong woman."

Seini could have said no to working with me on this first home. She worked long hours for little pay. She had trouble with her asthma in cold weather. If I wanted to feel guilty, I could have, with her bussing back and forth to work on cold days. She was just always there.

When we started our first home, much of it was ready, fire, aim. It seems like another lifetime, fourteen years ago. I'm more practical now than I was then because in order for us to do our work we have to look at licensing and finances and things like that. A lot has to be taken into consideration. But then it was an experiment and we did everything experientially. I'm glad Seini and I could share the experience together.

Filling the Well

Not only did residents arrive those first months, but so did a piano, a chair-lift, a business consultant, some volunteers, a media person, and a college class. One day I saw an ad on the grocery store bulletin board that said, "Piano, $400, restored upright. Delivered. Call Ed." I called Ed and bought the piano even though it was a little dilapidated. On a blustery winter day Ed and his brother backed his pickup truck up to the front door and hoisted the piano into the Rakhma living room. There was no bench. Ed promised he'd throw in a bench, but the piano bench that came a few days later looked like it had been in a fire, black and charred around the edges. I don't think we got the best deal, but anyway, it was important that we had a piano and music.

Music came before a chairlift, but it soon became clear that a two-level home without a chairlift kept potential residents from choosing Rakhma. "What if Mom can't make it up the stairs?" a daughter or son would lament. There were wonderful, empty bedrooms on the second floor that needed to be filled.

Inquiring into used chairlifts, I found one at a church for two thousand dollars. All Rakhma had was $350 in savings. A gentleman at the church suggested checking the bulletin board at a local hospital-home care equipment supply company. "Sometimes," he suggested, "people sell their used equipment that way." I marched over there and found a handwritten card advertising a chairlift. I called the number right away and went over to see it. The chairlift was on the stairway and it was just perfect. I asked the man how much he wanted for it. I can't remember the figure, but it was under a thousand dollars. I said all we had was three hundred and fifty dollars. He just looked at me. I told him about our first house that we were opening and finally he said, "Well, okay. You can have it, then, if you come and get it." A friend of a friend who had a truck picked it up and brought it over to Rakhma Home. No one can believe that we got a chairlift for that price.

Angels come in all forms. One day Marybeth called. She was an MBA student at St. Thomas University. She had found out about Rakhma through a board member, Chuck Smith, who worked as a student counselor at St. Thomas. She was interested in working with the elderly and wondered if she might be able to do an internship with Rakhma. I was thrilled, since my talents did not include putting together spreadsheets or collecting legal data. Marybeth's first priority was to write a business plan for Rakhma which included that kind of research. She would put the aim into my ready, fire, aim style.

Those months were so busy that I was exhausted most of the time. I didn't want to take time out to talk about business with Marybeth when there were residents to tend to and family members to meet with. Marybeth stood firm. "This has got to be done," she insisted. She settled me in a chaise lounge in the backyard one spring day before the mosquitoes were out. There we met for most of the day, Marybeth asking questions and taking notes. How do you do this? How do you do that? She wrote pages and pages out

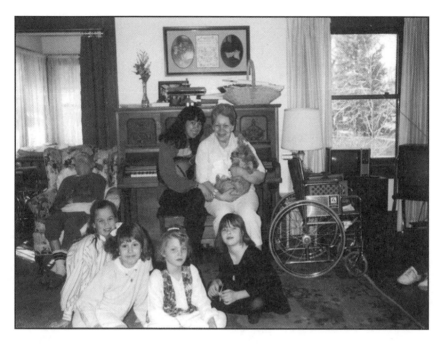

Our Rakhma piano

of which she would create a business plan describing organizational systems, capitalization plans, care plans, and staffing. "You mean I have that
much stuff in my head?" I exclaimed as the afternoon ended. "No wonder
I'm tired!"

Soon after Marybeth had launched into creating her business plan she
found out, due to some policy technicalities at St. Thomas, that she would
not be allowed credit for work done off-campus. Marybeth was so determined to stay involved with Rakhma that she transferred to Metropolitan
State University where she could design her degree with more flexibility.
After she completed the business plan for Rakhma, she got her MBA. Working with Rakhma redirected Marybeth's career. To complete the business
plan it was difficult to get certain types of information regarding housing
for the elderly. Licensing information in particular, according to Marybeth,

is the best kept secret in Minnesota. Much was wanted and needed in the area of housing for the elderly, and that is where she decided to specialize.

Thanks to Marybeth, the business-plan plate was spinning nicely, but what about publicity? The house was not full. I was living on money from refinancing my home supplemented by credit cards and a stipend from my former husband. I was working twenty-four hour shifts in the home while juggling the payroll records, management duties, staffing, intern supervision, fund-raising, resident recruitment, volunteers, and details of all sorts. The lack of a marketing budget combined with shyness about tooting my own horn kept Rakhma well hidden.

It took all I had to ask the pastor of a neighborhood church to allow me to share a little about Rakhma from the pulpit, but I was prodded by necessity. I was encouraged by the congregation's warm reception. When one speaks from the heart, people just naturally respond. Speaking publicly was hard in the beginning. However, as time went on, it was as if I stepped out of the way and just let my heart speak. I had become a vehicle for the vision of what is possible for the elderly.

I have known Lynn Baskfield now for more than twenty-five years. We co-owned a duplex together for ten of those years. We are like sisters, sharing a closeness and love that supports each other's lives, laughing and crying together over the years, watching each other's families grow and our work lives flower. Lynn has watched me develop the Rakhma vision, start my home-care service, and open all three of my homes. Lynn's mother, Dorothy, lived with dignity and love at Rakhma for the last two years of her life. It is time now to write this book, and I am lucky to have Lynn to do the actual writing.

Lynn did a little writing in the early days of Rakhma, too. She had experience with public relations efforts in her own business, so she started calling up local papers and pitching article ideas. Jim Martin from the *Metro Monitor,* a newspaper put out by the Twin Cities Metropolitan Council, came

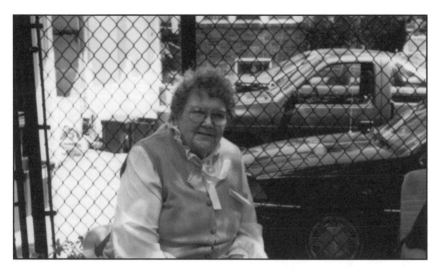

Evelyn Dorthea Hill

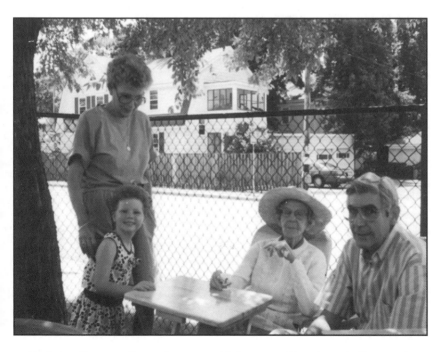

Barb Norling, our first volunteer, with her granddaughter Emily, Lynn's
mother Dorothy Baskfield and brother Jerry Baskfield

by to see the home and take pictures. He did a nice job telling the Rakhma story. From that first article, I got a number of encouraging phone calls. It felt really good to know that people were cheering me on. It gave me a much needed perspective. Log entries like this were not uncommon during that time:

> I was eating supper tonight, feeling wiped out from a confrontation with one of my staff. It isn't easy being boss and trying to watch over my business. I want things to go well for my residents, their families, my helpers, and myself. I want harmony. It doesn't always work that way. In the larger scheme of life, one conflict is small, though, compared to all the issues going on in the world like starvation, pollution, the aviation disaster that killed many Minnesotans this week. So God, I ask you to give me forgiveness, patience, and love.

And another entry, April 1985:

> Barb Norling, a volunteer, brought fresh fish that she fried for the ladies today. They all enjoyed it thoroughly. I had a lovely luncheon with one of our residents' daughters. We've been having a lot of phone calls from the article in the paper. I've had some great, supportive conversations. So many people out there.

And another April entry:

> Tuesday morning I arrived with Evelyn Dorthea Hill, a new helper at Rakhma I. Made a note to everyone, "Treat this helper well. She's somebody's mother—mine."

Helpers and volunteers came rather organically those first months. My mother had been cooking the Rakhma midday meal from my home and doing some office work from my sun-porch desk. For a while she helped out in the kitchen at Rakhma, too. My sister Betty Lou cooked from my

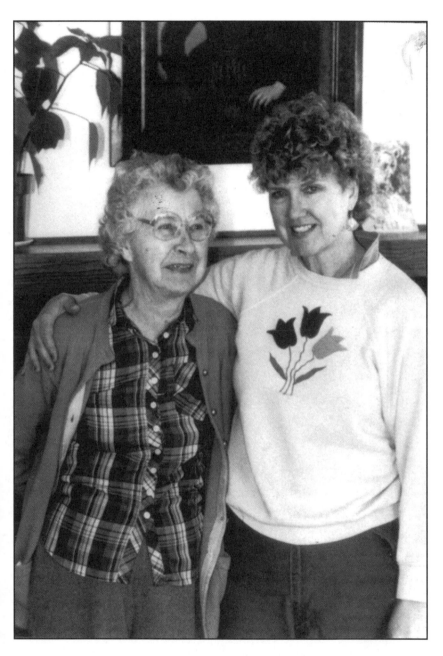

Hilda and Shirley, the first picture in the newspaper, *Metro Monitor*

home as well, sending heaping plates full of delectable goodies to the residents week after week.

Seini and I worked by ourselves for the first few months, keeping one staff person in the house at all times for the two original residents. When the number of residents increased from two to four after five months, I hired a night person. But it soon became apparent that two staff were needed days. Seini and I both worked days for a while. New staff came via friends of friends or friends of helpers. From the home-care service I had a nice network of people I knew to be competent and caring. I never advertised. They just came.

Volunteers also came through word of mouth. The first official volunteer was Lynn's sister, Barbara Norling, who came in to bake cookies, take Hilda for walks, shovel the sidewalk, or help with beauty-parlor day. Family of residents would come in and play the piano, an activity that almost always got the residents singing. That first article in the *Metro Monitor* put out the call for volunteers. Several people responded, one of them a handyman, Fred McGee, who stayed on for a long time providing much needed maintenance services.

They Will Come

After five months May and Gerry came to live at Rakhma.

As much as she wanted her mother to be able to live at Rakhma, May's daughter, Anita, held little hope for her adjustment there. May suffered from dementia which manifested in aggressive and belligerent behavior. Her doctor said a small, shared home probably would not work for someone with May's symptoms. After meeting with the family and taking her doctor's opinion into consideration, I devised a plan. If May could slowly develop a relationship with me and other staff she might better adjust to Rakhma Home. For the next three months, my helpers and I took May on outings and brought her to Rakhma for day care, preparing her to move in later, hopefully with few adjustment problems.

The first day I came to pick May up she was sitting by the front door with slippers on her lap. She was belligerent. Her house smelled of gas. A little looking around revealed that the oven was turned on, no flame. I got May dressed for an outing. We went out to lunch at a little nearby restaurant, then after a drive along the Mississippi River stopped for an ice cream cone. It turned out to be a fine day, similar to many others after it until it came time for May to move in.

May arrived at Rakhma permanently on April 22, 1985, amiable and humorous. After lunch she told me all about the charming man who sat next to her at the table. A baby came to visit that day and May, enamored, followed the little fellow all around the house. In the afternoon, though, she got anxious. I took her up to visit her room, to remind her that she had a room with her furniture right there. May became angry. She was incensed that her daughter Anita would leave her overnight. I listened, told her I understood, and she seemed to be reassured that she was welcome at Rakhma home. She was not going to be easy.

A note in the log:

When May arrived with her daughter, Anita, I wasn't sure what I was in for. I walked out to the car with them. May was mad at Anita for bringing her here. When she saw me she said to her daughter, "She's nicer to me than you!" She walked holding my hand, bopping Anita with a balloon she was carrying in the other hand. Anita slipped away while May was looking out the kitchen door at the blossoms on the trees.

Those first residents taught me that the first few days require a lot of time and energy to learn a person's patterns, yet the house needed to run as smoothly as possible so as not to disrupt the residents who are already comfortably settled. May's night pattern was peaceful. The second night was the only time she got up, and confused, got dressed and wandered into Hilda's room. Hilda said, "Where's your nightgown?" May replied, "I don't know."

Hilda said, "Maybe it's in your room. May said, "I don't know where my room is." Hilda said, "I must have another nightgown. Look in my closet. You can sleep in my bed."

So often, one resident will take another under their wing during that transition period when things are so unfamiliar. It's just a natural thing.

Beautiful, auburn-haired Gerry had spent many years doing everything in theater from making costumes to performing women's street theater. She often invited actors and actresses to elegant dinners at her Lake of the Isles home. She was especially fond of and involved with the nationally acclaimed Guthrie Theater. A vital woman with two college degrees and a myriad of other interests, her friends could barely keep up with her until Alzheimer's disease struck early in her fifties.

The changes in Gerry's behavior progressed rapidly. At night, through open curtains, a neighbor could see her pace back and forth past the window. During the day Gerry stopped wearing her flashy clothes and isolated herself at home. After she moved from her home to an apartment, a neighbor found her naked in the hallway, locked out of her living room. The neighbor called one of Gerry's three sons. It was clear something was drastically wrong. A thorough neurological exam indicated probable Alzheimer's disease. A second neurological exam yielded the same results. A nursing home, the doctors said, was the next step. Gerry's sons, grieving the loss of the mother they once knew and saddened by her losses as well, found themselves in a quandary: how to provide a life of dignity for Mom in the face of an undignified disease. They did not want their mom to go to a nursing home. Fortunately, around the time that all this was happening, they heard that Rakhma Home had recently opened.

Gerry came to Rakhma shortly after May arrived. When her sons toured the home, they brought her along. As they sat on the deck and talked, they agreed they all wanted her to live there. They mentioned that she had a golden retriever named Honey that had been in a kennel for three weeks

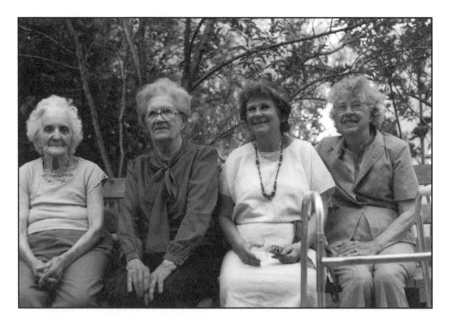

Our first four residents, Elan, May, Gerry, and Hilda

while Gerry was in the hospital being diagnosed. If she lived at Rakhma, they wanted to know, could she bring her dog? "I don't see why not," I heard myself say, "but we'll have to fence the yard."

I'll always remember the expression on Gerry's face when I said her dog could come. She was so happy she cried. A few weeks later the fence went up. It was one of those things we paid for monthly on the Sears card so we could have a place for Honey, the dog.

When Gerry first came, a lot of people came to visit her. The log book says: Gerry went with her friend Priscilla to Bachman's to buy some plants. She does need things to do. Gerry's son, Andy, took her to Dudley Riggs Comedy Club last night. She came home happy about 10:00. Her nights have been good since Sunday when Kelley gave her a foot rub and a backrub.

A month into having four residents, on May 28, 1985, I wrote:

I think sometimes I get real tired and frustrated, yet I am grateful
for the work we are doing.

Rakhma Home Prayer

I love you Elan, Hilda, May, and Gerry,
All my beautiful, wonderful helpers.
Mother/Father God
A special prayer for our house
A blessing I ask
That each day you help us
To be patient and loving one to another.
Remembering our purpose here on earth
Each person is as important as each other.
Help us to always remember that
and give us the strength and wisdom
and love we need.
P.S.: God, please continue to be an extra pair of eyes for us.
Thank you.
Amen.

Always Room for More

One room was still not filled. Until it was spoken for, I considered it a guest
room and encouraged family members from out of town to spend the
night. Gerry's son from California spent many nights there one summer, as
did one of Elan's daughters and other family members. "It's so nice to wake
up and be by Mother," the guests would say, crawling out from under a cozy
quilt to walk down the hall to their mother's room. Edith Stauffer, the woman
who inspired my overall philosophy with her Unconditional Love and For-
giveness workshops, came to Minneapolis to give a workshop and stayed
the night at Rakhma.

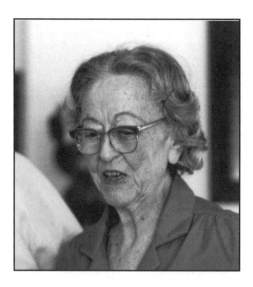

Our first Respite guest, Ella Winters

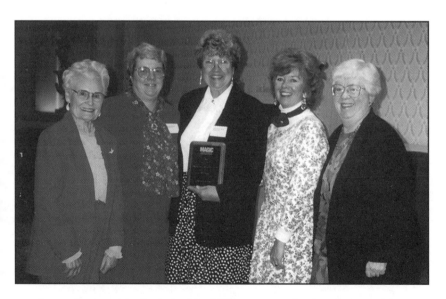

Accepting our Magic Award in 1993, an organizational recognition
award for Rakhma, Inc. At left is Edith Stauffer, who inspired me to
start Raklhma Home I. Pictured are (left to right), Edith Stauffer;
Shari Skally, nurse; Shirley Shaw, Director; Pam Boyce, volunteer and
Activities Coordinator; and Mary Ondow, board member.

It was a wonderful experience for me. Edith was so pleased to see this home manifest from her teachings that she wanted to do something for the ladies. A button had fallen off Hilda's sweater, so Edith sat with needle and thread in the sunroom and tightened up buttons. Then she washed the sweater in Woolite, and laid it out on the picnic table to dry. "Now I feel better," she said. That was part of her simple, inspiring spirit of service.

Part of the Rakhma vision in the beginning was to do respite care, where someone would come in for a short period of time if their caregivers needed a break, vacation, or hospital stay, then go back home again. In those beginning months a woman named Ella stayed for a few weeks. Up in years, bright, just a dear, she loved coming to the home, and it was a lot of fun for staff to have her. This was when there were only two residents. However, when Ella came back a year later after May moved in, her stay wasn't as enjoyable for her. May had a way of bluntly saying rude things to people. Strangers coming into the home are sometimes threatening and can bring out the worst side of the residents' personalities, just like what happens sometimes with little children. Now and then a resident can be pretty obnoxious.

I think it depends on the person who comes in and the people in the house. If you had someone coming in who wasn't difficult, and the people in the house were fairly easygoing, it could work. Respite in a home setting is needed. I love having a place in a home for people to use in this way. Just as in a family, you keep reaching out, extending hospitality, trying to include others as much as possible while at the same time creating a sense of safety and love within.

Despite setbacks, the Rakhma Home I took on a life of its own. The arms of family, I was to discover, have a very wide reach.

CHAPTER 3

Making Family

So many groups in the family soup
So many combinations
Might be people who look like you
Or they might be no relation
Birds of a feather they flock together
Yes, sometimes they do.
But if a little bird joins an elephant herd
Hey! That's a family too....
This is my home, these are my folks
These are our secrets and our habits
and our jokes.
We're free to be you and me.
And you and me, we're free to be a family.
—from the song "Free to Be a Family"
by Sarah Durkee
sung by Marlo Thomas

From the very first talks with Elan over lunch, honed by the months of home care shared with Doug and Lena, creating family has been a part of the Rakhma vision. Even when older people have family nearby, a sense of loneliness and isolation can permeate lives that have become more limited. Home is a wonderful place to be, yet friends have died, children are busy with their own lives, and time weighs heavily on a body that finds it harder to busy itself with the kinds of tasks running a house requires.

From the beginning, when a resident comes to Rakhma, we talk about family. We make sure he or she feels welcome, and we try to sustain that welcome with the little touches that make it safe to be here, to be yourself, to have things nearby that are familiar.

At Rakhma, family has many faces. It is the sons and daughters, relatives and friends of the Rakhma residents, their involvement in the resident's care and their own family dynamics. It is being a part of the world family of a culturally diverse staff and an ever-growing awareness of the interconnectedness of all life.

Strangers Become Family

When working with dementia, two things happen in the area of creating family. There is the coming together of unrelated people in the same household, who through the intimacy of daily living come to know and accept each other. And there is the confusion of the disease where often a resident thinks another resident is related in some way. For instance, Bowman Gravelle thought Norma Wiessner was his wife Annie. Norma didn't seem to mind, nor did her real husband Dick as he observed the consolation it provided each of them. Bowman even showed jealousy sometimes. Alice, a resident at the Rakhma Joy Home in Saint Paul, chats daily about others she thinks are relatives. Rakhma staff members realize that this sort of thing seems to bring the resident comfort, and take such departures from reality in their stride. To affirm another's reality is part of what loving is all about; it's just one more way of embracing a person as they are and giving them a place to express themselves.

Rakhma puts the person first and treats the condition, be it dementia, stroke, failing eyesight, or unsteady walking, as part of the person.

Many institutions focus on the condition. They don't purposely leave the heart and soul to atrophy, but that is what happens. Taking the time to get past the condition allows caregivers to focus on what the resident's life is all about. It's rather like mining for diamonds—it takes a lot of digging

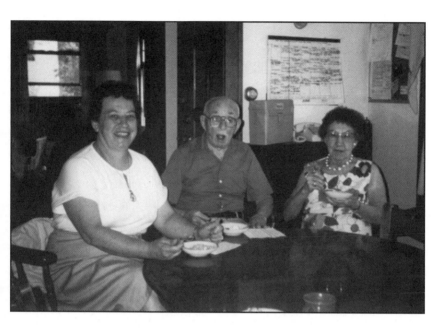

Coffee time at Rakhma Home I
Paul's daughter Elaine, Paul, and Paul's wife May

but there are brilliant points of contact with life that each resident has which, when discovered and polished, infuse old age with dignity and provide a true sense of belonging.

"That is Shirley's particular gift, paying attention," according to Judy Melinat, former assistant director of Rakhma. "The flu you can take care of, but the real point is that you're in the resident's home, their living space, and you are helping them make connections."

When Paul came to Rakhma he felt quite lost. "This is my house, isn't it?" he would say many times during the day.

"Yes, Paul. How do you know it's your house?" I would ask, triggering a pattern of response. Paul would look up, thinking. "I've got a bed upstairs…the furniture is familiar…there are good people here. Yes. It must be my house."

He didn't ask for his daughter or son, but he missed his wife of almost sixty years. He had memory loss. His wife had cancer and was sometimes unable to take care of him at home. After his daughter, Elaine, found Rakhma, she helped her mom move into an independent care apartment. Paul thought his wife was in a nursing home. "When are we going to be together?" he would lament. "The people here are nice, but I wish I could be with Mom."

Of course, no care model can take the place of one's own family. The losses that accompany becoming frail are real and can be debilitating in and of themselves. Rakhma doesn't pretend to be a substitute for what is missing. It simply includes it all, the joy and sadness, the fullness and emptiness—and listens.

"Rakhma was wonderful for Dad," according to Elaine. She tells how Paul came from Italy when he was a young boy, how vibrant he had been all his life, and how he stayed connected with life at Rakhma.

"Paul was a chef at Culbertson's Cafe until he retired at seventy-two. He was very proud of that. At Rakhma he could go out in the kitchen and cut up veggies and do other little things.

"And there was always music. One helper, Susie, had a way of getting Dad to play his mandolin. She'd put the mandolin in his hands and ask him to hold it for her. Pretty soon he'd start playing. He could play, but without the encouragement, he never wanted to. Another helper had a way of getting him to talk about the old days in Italy."

Paul was from Bardello, near Milan. He'd describe a bridge over a river where he used to go swimming, what his house was like, or other details of the town where he was born. When Elaine and her husband visited there, they found it exactly as Paul had described it. Upon seeing the photographs they took of his home in Italy, despite his memory loss, he lit up. "That's where I was born!"

Paul's boyhood dream was to become an architect. His father, who was working as a cement man in Fort Williams, Canada, wrote him that if he

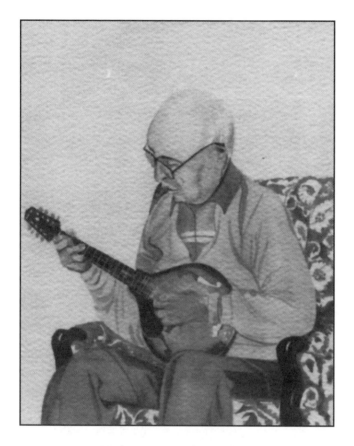

Paul Ferraaio with mandolin
pen and ink drawing by Elizabeth Manfrede

came to Canada, he would be able to attend the best schools. One day, as a cluster of family and friends was getting ready to set sail for New York, Paul heard there was room for one more passenger on the ship. He grabbed his bag and ran aboard. He was fourteen years old.

It is not clear how he made his way from New York to Fort Williams, but when he arrived there he found his Dad to be extremely fond of liquor and in need of a hod carrier. He worked for his father for some time until his father's friend, who felt he shouldn't be doing such heavy labor, sent him to Duluth, Minnesota, where another friend gave Paul a job in his restaurant.

As it turned out, the restaurant owner, too, was a drunk, often unable to produce the meals on his menu. Paul filled in for him many times, learning to cook in the process. He eventually opened his own Ideal Cafe in Duluth, saved his money, and brought his mother, brother, and two sisters to America.

Paul married and had a son. His first wife died when the boy was nine. After that Paul went to Minneapolis, where he remained in the restaurant business and married May, the waitress whom he missed so much at Rakhma.

However, having other people around to observe and form opinions about kept Paul interested and involved. Even the unusual things that are a part of living with dementia are stimulating for the residents. There is something outside of oneself to engage with. Another resident everyone called Grandpa didn't feel compelled to use the bathroom when he needed to urinate. Although under the close watch of staff, it would please him to find an alternative spot to relieve himself. One day Paul, half dozing, snapped to attention. "That old fart's peeing in the fireplace!" he exclaimed, incredulous. Sometimes life in your own living room is better than TV.

In spite of himself, Paul stayed connected. "I don't think it's possible to have a lot of places like Rakhma," Elaine says, "because there aren't enough people who care enough or understand dementia like Rakhma does."

Right now, Elaine is right. But part of the reason for writing this book is to encourage the development of more small homes that have a heart. Margaret Prod'Homme, R.N., of the Department of Neurology at the University of Minnesota Hospital and Clinic, cites the universal appeal of Rakhma's unique philosophy of unconditional love. Ms. Prod'Homme calls Rakhma a feeling-based model. "A lot of places don't have that," she says. "Rakhma does."

We all want our loved ones in a responsive environment. Dick Wiessner says of his wife Norma, "When I couldn't leave her alone at our house, I started looking for other alternatives. I had been actively involved at a nearby nursing home, one of the best in the country, for many years. I knew a lot about it, but it still wasn't good enough for Norma. Their care meets the high standards set by the Department of Health. Inspections require stainless steel counters, clean floors, good wiring, but they don't understand what the real needs of the individual are. People think the best way to care for the elderly is to put them in a beautiful, plush nursing home."

Norma spent her last years at Rakhma Joy Home where Dick was able to visit almost every day. But Dick's lifelong friend, Harry, was at the beautiful nursing home that Dick had been involved with as a volunteer. Recently, Harry was depressed, so Dick decided to take him out for a few hours. The nurse in charge that day advised against that because Harry had a mild cough. Also, she felt he was too depressed and tired to go out. She explained that the man Harry usually ate dinner with was grieving over the death of his wife and Harry was sad about that, too . Besides, Harry didn't get to rest in his bed that morning because maintenance people were working in his room.

Dick became frustrated as he evaluated the situation. The nurse was fully aware of Dick's lifelong relationship with Harry and his family. Since she also knew Dick had frequently taken Harry out of the home, she yielded to his persuasion.

"Here he was with all these people around him and he was lonesome. It's as simple as that. I took him to my house and fixed him a malted milk. We were only there about an hour, but it was familiar to him. In the institutional setting he was gradually losing all of his energy and interest in doing anything. There just wasn't enough stimulation and personal attention. I don't think he needed more rest. He needed more activity! Even though he was in one of the best nursing homes in the country, they were warehousing this guy. How can you do anything else with ten-to-one care ratio during the day? In some nursing home situations I've seen, there are ratios of up to sixty-to-one at night. You can't give individual attention; you just can't. A residential setting is far better than an institutional setting. In the home setting

the resident sees the kitchen, sees the groceries coming and going, and is
a part of daily living."

There are obstacles, but there is no reason why homes with a heart can't
thrive in every community. Later in the book we will look at the roadblocks
to creating such homes and make suggestions for paving the way.

Family as Never Before

Rakhma creates family in a way that some people have never experienced
it before.

Sylvia was a Finnish immigrant who celebrated her one hundredth birthday on January 31,1995, and died two days later. She was one of the first
residents at the Joy Home in St. Paul. She had been declared incompetent
by the courts and was assigned a conservator, Pat Murphy.

When Sylvia was a girl of nine, several of her cousins were leaving Fin-
land for the United States when one suddenly got cold feet and refused to
go. On a moment's notice, Sylvia was substituted for her cousin, torn from
her family and homeland, and was put on a ship bound for America. Here
she developed a strong work ethic and learned to take care of herself.

A machinist by trade, Sylvia was a fiercely independent soul. She owned
a cozy house on Cedar Lake Road in north Minneapolis. She didn't marry
the man she loved early in life because he couldn't get work. Much later she
became friends with a woman with whom she lived for thirty years.

At ninety-two, when she couldn't get around anymore, she was placed
in a nursing home not far from her house. There, confined to a wheelchair,
she became depressed and extremely unhappy.

Her conservator, Pat, was working at the time for a corporate elder care
system. Large and lovely, her company was looking to expand its services
to include smaller, homelike settings in their care options. As part of her job
Pat was researching existing shared homes when she came across Rakhma.
Very impressed, she knew Sylvia would thrive here and made arrangements
for her to move.

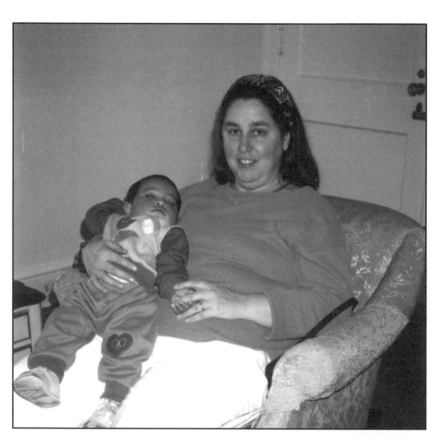

Judy Melinat and Cilla

Sylvia had legs that shouldn't have been able to walk. The doctor could move her leg bones laterally out from the knee joint, but within a week of coming to Rakhma, Sylvia engineered her way all over the house using only a walker. She fell a lot, but she knew she would fall. She just laughed and with help got up again. It was much better for her than being restrained. Her vision was so poor that her glasses looked like Coke bottles, and you had to yell into her hearing aid to make yourself understood.

Sylvia read the obituaries in the *Star Tribune* every day just to make sure she wasn't dead. Then she'd laugh.

"She was our grandma in the house," says Judy, our former Joy Home manager and later assistant director. "We moved her furniture into the double room on the first floor where she loved to sit by the window and watch me garden. She liked to give me advice through the open window."

Certain staff members became her special friends. She was racially intolerant, putting some of the black caregivers through hell until she got to know them. "It's an amazing thing that they bore up under that," muses Judy, "but they came through."

"She loved people despite her racism," observes Judy. "She needed people and made the place her home. She got a big kick out of people and interacted with everyone with a real open heart. She always gave backrubs and foot rubs to staff."

When other residents were sick, Sylvia would make little visits. Sylvia had some confusion about who were women and who were men. One very feminine helper, Lynn, was always a boy to Sylvia, and black people were always men. But she enjoyed talking to residents who figured she wasn't senile, just hard of hearing. One resident, Pauline, could be quite condescending. When she was, Sylvia delighted in making cracks about Pauline's character.

"Sylvia was really a free spirit," recounts Judy, who has an understanding that sees beneath a feisty exterior and mirrors her soul. "We became friends, but she had trouble with me because she saw me as the boss here in the house, and to her the boss means no freedom. She valued freedom for herself and others.

"Next to freedom, her other two big loves were a little cup of coffee with lots of sugar, and pickled herring, not necessarily at the same time."

Like Paul, Sylvia could always differentiate between being at Rakhma and being at her home on Cedar Lake Road, where she could have coffee with her next door neighbor, Elsie. Though disabled by stroke, Elsie sometimes came to Rakhma to share a little cup of coffee with lots of sugar, thanks to the rides provided by conservator Pat.

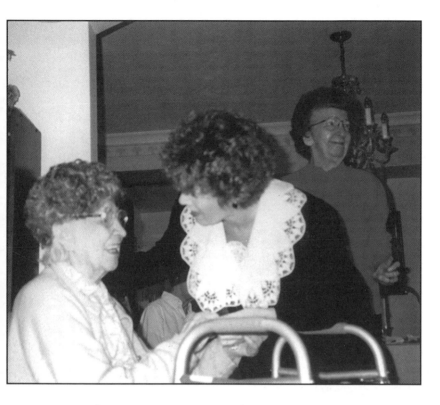

Sylvia, conservator Pat Murphy, and friend Elsie

"This is your home," Judy would tell Sylvia. "I'm so glad you're here. It isn't home, we know, but it's the next best thing. We love you here."

Pat felt that helping Sylvia reconnect with her Finnish heritage would be another way to create family for her. Pat's extensive research brought forth names of long-lost Finnish relatives. Pat got in touch with them, and they sent letters and photos to Sylvia. Although she blustered with annoyance that this had happened without her knowledge, Sylvia nevertheless sat down every few days with Rakhma helpers to pore over the pictures and hear again the news of the family with whom ties had been severed early in life.

Pat's commitment all along was to communicate Sylvia's real self to others and to make a connection with people who could appreciate who

Sylvia was. "And we really did," affirms Judy. "You couldn't help but like or dislike Sylvia. She loved to have people sit on her lap. She was like a Zen master. She would zone in on your soul. If your soul didn't interest her, you were not in the queen's good graces."

As a conservator, Pat's clients rarely have family involved in their care or may not have had involvement with family for many years. Says Pat, "Rakhma is the home they never had."

Others, like Norma Wiessner, come from close-knit families and have been cared for for a long time by a spouse or other family member. Alzheimer's disease involves the family in ways that only a person who has been through caring for someone who has it can understand. There may be a long period of care giving, many unsung heroic acts, and a struggle with the inevitable step of finding an alternative that is the next best thing to one's own family.

Caring for Alzheimer's Disease at Home: The Family Dilemma

"It's easily described but not easily understood until you experience it," says Dick Wiessner as he talks about caring for his declining wife alone at home for six years prior to her moving to Rakhma. "In the early stages as they are losing it mentally, they also become physically dependent. They follow you around like you have a trailer hooked to you. They cling. It's hard to find the right words. The only way anyone really ever knows the difficulty in caring for someone like that is to just do it."

Norma and Dick had planned to spend their retirement years working with children and traveling. Dick was fifty-six and Norma fifty-four when dementia of the Alzheimer's type was diagnosed. Their bright, comfortable future flickered like a candle in the wind, then darkened into a time of grief and anguish.

Although women normally live longer than men and are four times more likely than men to be long-term caregivers as their husbands or parents decline, Dick emphasizes that a lot of men become caregivers too, do a good

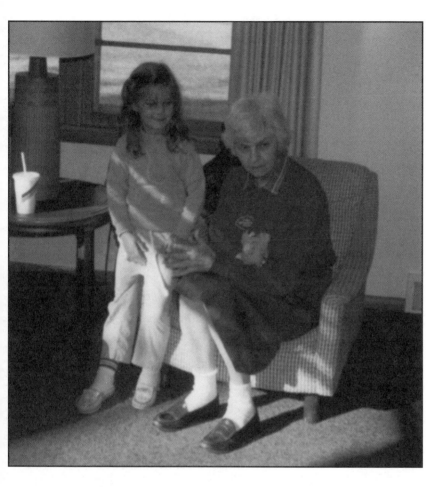

Norma Wiessner and granddaughter Emily

job, and have a lot of the same concerns. It's tough for men, he says, because
not only do they face the challenges of a future that includes Alzheimer's
disease, if they haven't been domestic before, they need to learn to cook,
do laundry, and juggle things on the home front.

"I hauled so many Campbell Soup labels to church for the label drive
that they got concerned," says Dick. "Then I discovered frozen TV dinners.

I wasn't too dumb to cook, just too busy. When you have someone so dependent, you don't have time or energy for much else but to keep up with them."

As Norma's disease progressed, Dick turned for help to the Alzheimer's Disease Association, which was still very new.

Hilda Pridgeon staffed the tiny Minneapolis office alone. The only printed information available was what she ran off on a copy machine. Dick, on his own, found a number of people to talk to—including a lawyer—and received this advice:

1. Get divorced. This disease will eat up all your assets.

2. It's going to get worse. Figure out what you're going to do with the rest of your life.

Later, Dick described it this way: "You have two problems: the person with Alzheimer's disease, and the caregiver who goes along from day to day until he or she is no longer able to function. The caregiver's breakdown comes months and months before other family members really know what's going on. You're dealing with fatigue and disenchantment with life. You're discouraged and you don't know where to go or what to do. You're around people who act like they care for you, but they don't really understand. They look in on you.

"At the end of each day you reflect back and think, 'I got through the day all right. I can manage this.' The next day, however, gets slightly worse. You repeat this process until gradually you're done in. Every day you cope until it isn't possible anymore."

Despite the enormous challenges, Dick wasn't ready to have Norma live elsewhere. He and Norma had a large stately home with a big backyard in St. Paul. Dick thought it would lend itself to becoming a cooperative day-care center for others in the same boat. The house could be a gathering place for two to six people with Alzheimer's disease. A couple of caregivers could stay with them for the day while the others had a little escape. As a lifelong resident of the area, Dick knew a lot of people and found fifty families within four miles of his home. This is the letter he wrote to them:

This letter is addressed to individuals with addresses in the vicinity of my home who are known to have indicated an interest in the care of someone with AD or a related disorder.

For five years now I have been taking care of my wife at home while she has been steadily declining as a result of AD. She is now 61 years old.

It is difficult to take her with me every time I leave the house. However I do not want to consider nursing home placement at this stage. As an alternative, I would like to consider sharing care time with one or more others who may have a similar situation. We have a large home, easily accessible, near Macalester College, which would lend itself to a cooperative arrangement of some sort. It may be practical to engage custodial or even professional assistance from outside part of the time.

I would like to hear from others who may consider a cooperative care arrangement.

Dick got a lot of calls and a few letters back, but the initiative, he says, didn't work.

One couple was in their eighties. The woman had Alzheimer's disease, the man was going blind. Their daughter and son visited them from time to time and felt they were getting along okay. Dick received a series of distressed phone calls from the man, usually about six in the evening, which is often a difficult time for Alzheimer's victims. "She's awful," the husband would say. "She can't tell the difference between salt and sugar. She gets so demanding she won't let me go get the mail."

Dick knew this was a desperate situation and that these people needed more than day care help. He called the daughter to alert her to the scope of the problem, but as is so often the case with family members who do not live in the household, she still was not concerned. He finally called the man's church for help.

Another man in his late seventies lived two blocks away.

"The guy started calling from his apartment. I'd hold the phone for forty-five minutes and let him spill the beans. He had owned his house and had it all paid for, but when his wife entered a nursing home, he soon depleted all his assets caring for his spouse who had Alzheimer's. He did what you call spending down, paying for nursing home costs. He got a new mortgage, then a second mortgage.

"Finally he had no assets. At that time state law allowed you to retain $10,000 in assets and income up to $575 per month. He sat in a little apartment over on Grand Avenue. He drove his old car until repair costs exceeded its value. He was a candidate for suicide. He became a ward of the state himself. That's what convinced me to get a divorce. The liquid assets went to Norma. I kept the physical assets."

Dick's situation was different than many. Being only fifty-six years old, he was physically and mentally competent to take charge of caring for his wife. He was independent enough in his job so that he could phase out and retire early. He needed to be with Norma one hundred percent of the time and prided himself on being highly independent and self-sufficient. He was a strong man, yet even the strongest wear down. He describes that process:

"The fatigue becomes unbearable. Whenever I had to go somewhere even for a short time, I had to take her with me. If I went to the grocery store, I had to take her in. If I left her in the car, she would get out and walk away. One time I found her outside a large shopping center following a woman, asking her, 'Who am I? Who am I?' The woman was mad. She wanted that crazy person out of there.

"Another time when Norma got away I found her three or four blocks from our house. One time in the later stages of her disease, she had gotten out of the car a half mile from home and I drove around looking for her. Not being able to find her, I got so frustrated I just got in the car and went home. I was almost wishing she'd get hit by a train. Strangely enough, when I got home, she was there."

Like so many caregivers, Dick hung on longer than he should have. When you are in the thick of the situation, it is easy to go well beyond the

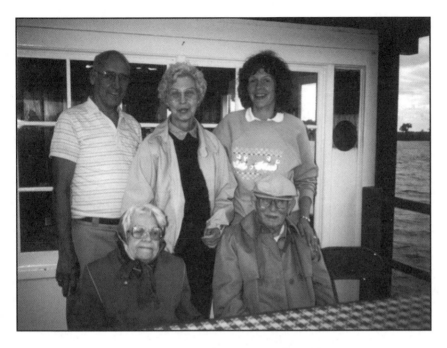

An outing on Lake Minnetonka with
Dick, Norma, June (back, left to right), Betty, and Paul (front)

point where you can give the individual the best care. When the caregiver gets to the point to where that's all they're doing, there is no life left.

"That's when I got into trouble. Even the church faded into the background, a church we'd been active in for forty years.

"The church said, 'Here's an in-house project.' They made lists of who would bring us hotdish. Some came. Some didn't. Then the project petered out. When we couldn't participate anymore, it was as if we just disappeared. Couples like that become extremely isolated. There is nothing you can do. It becomes a chore for friends to be friends.

"Then we got up one morning and after dressing her, Norma looked at me and said, 'Where's Dick?' The Alzheimer's Association said this would happen, but you can't really be prepared. From then on it happened more and more often. 'Who do you think I am?' I'd ask her. How could my wife of forty years not know me? Apparently I was now a substitute for whatever was left from the past."

Not enough other younger couples responded to Dick's day-care letter. The Alzheimer's Association started looking for other resources for him, but the progression of Norma's disease was devastating. "I couldn't do it anymore," relates Dick. "For a long time I hated to pass up a good-looking bridge abutment. Investigators would say a tire blew out. He lost control."

Nevertheless, looking for more resources was the trigger that got Dick together with me. I was willing to take Norma for day care at Rakhma. It was Dick's initial contact with a noninstitutional setting.

"I was not willing to put Norma in an institutional setting. It's difficult for a spouse to leave family in a nursing home. During those first six or seven months of knowing Shirley, I got a lot of relief. Rakhma was a day care for Norma. I'd drive up to the house, she'd see the chain-link fence around the backyard. She couldn't wait to get in there.

"People with AD know they're not up to speed. They're losing it, can't control it anymore. They see other people's irritation and feel their antagonism. They withdraw. But put two people together with dementia, they're perfectly fine. Norma was happy a lot of months in day care at Rakhma."

The crash came one morning when Dick had just gotten Norma out of bed and ran to answer the phone. He had helped her to the bathroom, but had not seated her on the toilet. In the time it took to go to another room to answer the phone, tell the caller he couldn't talk right then, and get back to Norma in the bathroom, she had had a bowel movement in the bathtub. Dick sat with his head in his hands. Norma didn't even know the difference between the tub and the toilet. It just kept getting worse. How could he keep going? A few minutes later I called, and he poured out his story.

"I'm coming over," I said gently but firmly. "I think it's time for Norma to come and stay with us for a few days." Dick knew by my voice that if he tried to stop me, I'd come anyway. "Get me a suitcase, Dick," I said quietly as I walked in. I packed some things and took Norma by the hand, helped her into my old blue Buick, and drove her to her new home at Rakhma.

Family Systems

Residents come to Rakhma bringing not only their clothes, furniture, and Alzheimer's disease, but they come with their family system in tow as well. As in Dick's case, there might be a burned-out caregiver and supportive children cooperating to make the transition from living at home to living in a shared home.

In other cases, there may be differing opinions about care, strong emotional ties or lack of them, unresolved or dysfunctional communication patterns, feelings about aging, overwhelming sibling relationships, or grief that make taking care of the resident a piece of cake compared to dealing with the family. Yet families are an integral part of elder care and must be given lots of room to design plans and participate in the care of their loved one. The ideal of the geriatric Waltons has given way at Rakhma to a more practical approach born of on-the-job training along with ongoing education in working with families. And because each family is different, bringing a mix of dynamics unlike any other family, the training goes on, somewhat like improvisational dance. You train the body to respond to the the music, whatever that may be.

Many things go on in a family. Let Mom be at home a while longer, one family member insists. Another wants to try a different setting, perhaps look at independent living. One wants to see her in Rakhma Home where she would have company and the family wouldn't have to worry about her wandering off and getting lost.

Shari Skally, our nurse and intake person until 1996, had gentle ways of nudging families into a unified decision-making process. Sometimes she would conduct a series of meetings by phone or face to face with one person, with a family sub-group, or with the whole family.

When Rakhma was new, I took to heart the advice of a speaker at the Minnesota Alzheimer's Association annual meeting: If you can understand the family system and accept it, your work with the resident will be much easier because there is no family system that's the same.

When I heard that, I said, "Phew, we don't have to work so hard." Working with the family system, we can look more clearly at what is possible for the resident, given everyone who is involved. Some families are exceptional at working together and working with us, creating the kind of care that goes beyond what we could do ourselves. Others are at odds with us or with each other. When there isn't a lot of cooperation, now we try to determine who are the main decision makers and let them plod through the family system. And then saying the Serenity Prayer a lot helps too!

"God, grant me the serenity to accept the things I cannot change, to change the things I can, and the wisdom to know the difference."

When it works, it works well. For instance, there is one resident who wanted to be in charge of when she bathed and washed her hair. The difficulty was that she did these things all too infrequently, remaining blithely unaware of her ripe condition.

She would, with resistance, let staff bathe her, but she wouldn't let anyone wash her hair, insisting that she had it done at the hairdresser, which of course never happened. The woman had a granddaughter who was quite close to her. The house manager called the granddaughter and said, "We have a problem." Her granddaughter stepped in with a brilliant solution—give Grandma a Christmas gift certificate for a weekly shampoo and set at the nearby hairdresser's. The gift was graciously accepted. Since she's had her hair done regularly, Grandma has been less snappish and feels better about herself.

It wasn't unusual to see this same woman wearing her long-sleeved black angora sweater on a humid July day. She would not part with her winter clothes and made herself miserable wearing them all summer. Again, the granddaughter was asked to come to the home and help. On a day when all the residents were at Perkin's Pancake House for lunch, the granddaughter sorted her grandma's drawers, leaving only the summer things. She let her Grandma know later that she took the winter things to the dry cleaners and tucked them away for next season.

Though it was not quite the truth, it gave Grandma some peace of mind, knowing that someone she trusted had taken care of her things.

Even though the decision to move someone out of their home is a hard one for families, the move, after a time of transition, can change the family dynamic, many times for the better. It's easier to make Mom or Dad more comfortable in a residential setting than at their own home, simply because there is more help and more attention. The everyday things are taken care of. The support systems are in place. When responsibilities no longer cause them concern, residents are often more available for personal relationships.

Mom or Dad can become easier to deal with and at some point relationships with family members may get better. One daughter of a Joy Home resident said, "Thank you for helping me get my mom back again. We have a relationship we haven't had for many years."

Through these mundane kinds of situations, breakthrough work is being done in Rakhma living rooms and kitchens, at the shampoo bowl and the storage closet, at meetings around the dining-room table with families, over the phone with sons and daughters.

Alzheimer's disease poses more questions than answers at this stage.

How do we provide dignified care with a heart in a homelike setting to people with dementia? How do we involve families so that the care is a seamless team effort?

It's an ongoing educational process. Anything we learn that works we can certainly suggest to other families. And we're always learning.

Each home has its own home manager and staff which brings a certain energy to the house, making up its own "family" system.

When a new resident comes aboard, family members meet the helpers and the other residents, and are encouraged to get to know how the house functions and how people interact. Conversely, when a new resident comes in, the nurse and I give staff as much information as possible about the resident and family they will be working with.

House managers say that before family and residents, their hardest job is managing staff. So all of the systems must be managed, keeping in mind that the heart of care is the residents.

Residents, even with behavior problems, even with family systems that are difficult to work with, are embraced by the Rakhma philosophy of love. Each person has room to be themselves. Each person's inherent beauty shines through.

Just Dorothy

Lynn's mother, Dorothy, lived on Blaisdell Avenue in a small apartment just a block from her house. When her memory began to slip—though quite gradually at first—it became more and more difficult for her to do many little tasks that had always come easily. Lynn checked in on her almost every day, sometimes to eat chocolate ice cream with her out of pink Melmac bowls, sometimes to do her taxes or balance her checkbook.

On the short walk over to Dorothy's one May day after an envelope of canceled checks had come in the mail, the sun cloaked Lynn in its warmth after a long, gray Minnesota winter. Robin song carried lightly through the branches of the budding elms. She took a deep breath, drinking in the sweetness, the freedom of the moment. She knew her mother's small apartment would be hot, and that as much as she wanted to help, it was not easy being with her. Their relationship had improved over the years, but even when Dorothy was well, the two of them thought very differently. Their conversations aborted like so many liftoffs at Cape Canaveral, and Lynn wanted to travel the galaxy with her mom.

They remained earthbound. Now with Dorothy's advancing Alzheimer's disease, it was like wearing lead shoes. "Are my checks all right?" "When do we pay taxes?" "I should invest in something different." "I can't invest

in something different. The bank
may fail." "Have I paid the rent?"
"Are my checks all right?" she
would ask over and over again.

As usual, Lynn piled the
checks on her mother's table, got
out the calculator, and started sort-
ing. Dorothy sat on her beloved
green French provincial couch
watching and waiting. As much as
she tried to sit quietly, she couldn't
help asking her questions. Lynn
would always answer briefly and
as politely as she could, although
she knew her impatience came
through as she scribbled things in
and crossed things out. She wanted
to concentrate on the numbers and
finish the task at hand.

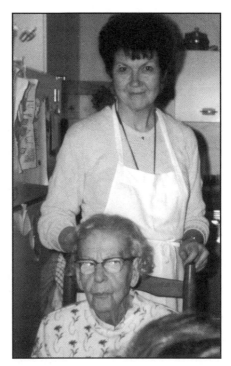

Lynn Baskfield with mother Dorothy,
doing hair

"Are my checks all right?"
asked Dorothy tentatively.

Unlike all the other times, all the months and years before when Lynn,
despite her love, was driven crazy by her mother's ways, that ordinary, repetitive moment opened between them like a flower as she glanced up from
her work to answer her mom's question. She looked into her mother's eyes
and saw her face as if for the first time. She was not the Dorothy Lynn
thought she knew—not the person who asks tedious questions; not her
mother who did or did not do all the things she thought a mother should do;
not a woman of eighty-four, someone with whom she didn't see eye to eye.
She was just Dorothy. And she was so beautiful.

There was no need at that moment to balance the checkbook.

"Mom, I want to thank you for all you've done for me," Lynn heard herself say from the very core of her being. Dorothy had gotten up from her chair, but stopped short on her way to her tiny kitchen. Though partially blind, she looked directly at Lynn.

"Lynn, I love you so much. I wish I could have done more."

"Mom, you gave me my life. What more could you have done?"

Lynn had been the blind one all these years and now she saw.

There was nothing more to do.

Dorothy held out her hands to her daughter. They sat down together on the green couch for the rest of the afternoon. She told Lynn stories about growing up in St. Paul and about Lynn's father who had died when she was a child and about how she still missed the man who had been her one love.

After that nothing changed that you could see. Lynn's mother was still her mother, funny, stubborn, forgetful, and asking the same questions over and over. And Lynn still got impatient with her sometimes. But in that one moment, everything changed. In that one moment Lynn knew who her mother was, and even as she became more frail and dependent in her illness, Lynn was able to be with just Dorothy all the rest of her life. And she was so beautiful.

Lynn began to see how gracious she was and how very generous. She saw past her mom's fierce independence and discovered her soft vulnerability. She saw how not being able to express her love and verbalize her feelings had cost her mother a great deal. She saw that she loved, nevertheless, as fully and fiercely as she knew how.

Dorothy was a devout Catholic with an unflagging faith in God. She was a graceful lady who loved to dance. She had good friends with whom she played bridge before her memory loss made it too hard to keep track of the cards. She was like a second mother to Lynn's children, taking care of them while she, a single mom, worked, went to college, and occasionally traveled.

After Dorothy moved to Rakhma, Lynn and her sister Barb found a log of baby-sitting hours she had kept with dates and times and totals for each month, each year. As her memory loss progressed she kept track of things by writing notes her daughters found—about doctor's appointments and what the doctor said, about symptoms she was having, about financial concerns, about when she bought groceries.

Brother Jerry, Barb, and Lynn sat down with Dorothy one day to discuss, while she was still able to do so, where she would choose to live if she couldn't stay in her apartment.

She refused to talk about it, saying she would stay where she was until she died. That was her plan. The "kids" tried to explain how they would like that too, but if something should change, wouldn't she want to have a say in what happened to her and not feel as if she were put somewhere by others. "Over my dead body," was her response to that idea.

Dorothy's memory loss kept getting worse. Lynn found herself exhausted and not really knowing why. As Dick Wiessner described earlier, Alzheimer's creeps up on you. You become more and more accustomed to filling in for the person who can no longer take care of daily matters and before you know it, you have little time of energy to conduct your own life. She needed some time away, so Barb invited their mother to stay at her house while Lynn spent some time with a friend in the Colorado Rockies.

Shortly after Lynn returned home, Dorothy started talking about things she had never talked about before. "Are you happy?" she asked on the way home from a Mother's Day gathering at Barb's house. "I want you to know that you were special to me. You came so late in my life." A little later that evening she said, "You were always different than the others. Deep. I didn't always connect the circle, so I didn't understand the poems and the stories you wrote. But they were beautiful. I am proud of you."

Later that night Lynn rushed Dorothy to the emergency room. She had been running through the halls of her apartment building knocking on doors and yelling, "Call the police. Call the police."

"I haven't lived here in years," she told the ambulance driver, "and my daughter is trying to hurt me."

It is hard to know just when it is time for a loved one to leave their home. "Do we wait until she falls down and breaks something?" we ask ourselves. "Do we wait until she burns herself on the stove she forgot to turn off? Do we take action before something drastic happens?" After this incident Lynn and her family knew this was it. As soon as Rakhma had an opening, Dorothy's children arranged for her to live there. They knew it was a place where the caregivers would appreciate "just Dorothy" every day.

One of the nice things about Rakhma is that you can stop over any time. The first week Dorothy was there, Lynn would go over and tuck her into bed at night. After she settled in, Lynn didn't stay until bedtime but felt free to ring the bell around 7:30 or 8:00 in the evening with ice cream from the Tom Thumb down the street. Some residents might still be up watching TV in the living room or reading the paper. Some might be going about their bedtime rituals with the help of staff. Lynn and her mom would go upstairs where Dorothy's room was. The second-floor kitchen, dining room, and living room of the Rakhma duplex were little used, and even though Dorothy never really remembered where she was, it was a good place to enjoy a visit. Most evenings, Helen, whose room was also on the second floor, was bustling around in her yellow cotton robe and fuzzy slippers.

"Helen, would you like to join us for ice cream?" Lynn would ask.

"Oh, my, yes, if it wouldn't be too much trouble, I'd love to! What kind is it?"

"It's chocolate, Helen."

"Chocolate? I love chocolate. It's my favorite." And Helen would sit down to eat with mother and daughter, the ice cream sweet and cold and real on their tongues.

Family Members Include Others

When Elan's daughter came to visit, she always brought enough Danish and doughnuts for everyone. She might have been anyone's daughter coming in the door, greeting people, bringing something to dunk in the coffee always freshly brewed in a pot in the kitchen. In a state of dementia, a resident might look up and think Elan's daughter was their own wife or daughter. It didn't matter. She was there to greet and hug them, and when she left, the residents felt like they had a special visit from family.

Sometimes family members get more than they bargained for when they come to visit, like a car full of instant grandmothers. One particularly beautiful day Dorothy's son, Jerry, stopped over to take her for a ride around Lake Harriet. Dorothy, feeling particularly gracious, invited Hilde and Helen to come along. Before he knew it, Jerry had two more passengers eager for some outdoor fun.

"It was like that scene in *One Flew Over the Cuckoo's Nest* when everyone is out on the raft," recalls Jerry. "Hilde was too cold. Helen was too warm. Mom was just right."

Hilde, in her soft voice, chatted on about her granddaughter who owns the bakery on 36th and Bryant. Dorothy, wringing her hands, worried the whole time about where she would sleep that night. Helen, enjoying the joggers as they sped past the budding trees that overhung the rippling lake, exclaimed at how lovely it all was.

"Everyone seemed to enjoy the trip immensely," said Jerry. "As I drove along it occurred to me that being in that car was a lot like life—no one seems to listen to each other anyway!"

In Jerry's case, somewhat to his surprise, his mom did the inviting. In other cases, family members intentionally invite other residents along on outings because they find their mom or dad feels more secure and content. Sally Flax's mother, Isabel, in the beginning wanted to go home with her daughter and live there. After staying at Rakhma for a while, she became more anxious when at Sally's. With another resident along, Sally found that Isabel was more relaxed, especially at that sundowner time after dinner. When they went back to Rakhma, Isabel was glad to be home and to have a companion that stayed as Sally waved goodbye.

When Dorothy got so that taking her out, especially to family gatherings or crowded places, made her so confused and agitated that it was no fun to go, her family brought the party to her. The upstairs kitchen, dining room, and living room were little used during the day by residents, who usually gathered on the downstairs couch and overstuffed chairs where it was easy to watch household goings on, see who came to the door, and smell dinner cooking on the stove. The family had Mother's Day and two Christmas parties upstairs. In came the Crockpots, the crackers, and the cakes. The Rakhma staff contributed coffee, tea, and trimmings to the festivities, and on Christmas, dishes from around the world.

Everyone who wanted to trekked upstairs, some with help, to join the fun. Dorothy, always the gracious hostess, remained queenly and polite, even though she was sure she was on a ship to Norway.

Every month Rakhma has a potluck dinner at one of the homes to keep family and friends involved in a social way. Everyone brings something; there is good conversation, music, and sometimes even dancing. Helpers bring their children to visit. Residents feel connected to little ones; occasionally they even get possessive and don't want to share them with anyone else. Helpers' children come to read, walk, and play checkers with the residents. One eleven-year-old sits on the piano bench and reads out loud to the many residents who enjoy little children's stories. Sometimes the kids play ball with residents or give musical recitals.

When babies visit, faces light up. Residents remember their own baby from their own family; maybe this is their baby. Grandpa (the same Grandpa who peed in the portico), a short little man, would slip right down on the floor off his chair and play with toddlers who pulled his beard and made everyone laugh.

The World Family

Rakhma is a reminder that no matter how small you are, one voice can make a difference. A local nonprofit with three small homes, Rakhma embodies a consciousness which acts locally and thinks globally. Staff members come from all over the world—places like Cambodia, Liberia, and Tonga, to name a few.

As in a nuclear family, each person brings diverse viewpoints and ways of doing things, but unlike most nuclear families, each person opens a window to a different corner of the world. Such diversity among the staff constantly reminds me that we don't always hear or do things the same way. Perhaps our way is not always the best way. I think about the wisdom that each person brings. It's interesting, but it's not always easy. There have to be policies and procedures, but the heart that Rakhma provides withers when policies, not people, become primary.

Many helpers are relatives or friends from the same community in their homeland. Being in daily contact with people of other cultures and colors is not an experience most of the residents had before living in Rakhma's homes. There are so many beautiful faces. Our residents have dementia, but in daily life, when staff members talk about what's happening with relatives in Liberia, for instance, it brings a momentary awareness to residents, an expanded view of family and a window to the world. I can't even imagine some of the hardships our helpers have gone through. Many of them have been uprooted and unable to see even their spouses or children.

Before the war in Liberia, Martha Nehwah came to the United States for a visit to a relative to see if this might be a place she could bring her family to live. Her husband cautioned, "If war breaks out, don't come back. The children need one parent to be safe and to provide for them." While she was here war did break out. She called her husband on the phone. "If you come back, we could all be killed," he said, "or we would have to break up our family and go into hiding."

Crying into the phone, Martha pleaded to come back. Her husband said, no, speak to the children. The children said, "Mom, you have to stay there so we can come to be with you." Martha could barely function, yet she worked two to four jobs at a time, keeping only money for food and rent. The rest of the money she sent to her family.

Seven years later her children were given permission to leave Liberia rather suddenly and Martha needed six thousand dollars to fly them to Minneapolis. Since she had bought a small house and a car in anticipation of this moment, the bank would not float another loan for the airfare. Their visas gave her only a small window of time to get her children here, and they were about to run out.

Martha found people who were willing to charge the tickets on their credit cards, with the stipulation they be paid back in a month. The children came with only the clothes they were wearing. Martha turned to me for help.

I appealed to friends at two churches for loans. Both St. Luke's Presbyterian Church in Minnetonka and the Wayzata Community Church came forth with the money to have six of the children over. Wayzata Church also had beautiful people like Jan Reardon donating clothes and bedding.

Even though Martha and her children started out sleeping three to a bed, she said she hadn't slept so peacefully in years.

Martha visited both of the churches later with her children to thank the congregation. The children sang for them. There weren't many dry eyes afterward.

Rakhma Peace Home manager Winnie received news that her mother, Florence, was run over by an army convoy truck on April 19, 1996, during an attack on Monrovia, Liberia, where she lived. Fleeing the attack, she had already safely crossed the road over which the convoy passed, but was killed when she ran back to save two frightened children who were still on the other side.

Florence died as she had lived. Although she had six children of which Winnie was the oldest, everyone was her family in her eyes. She was a nurse by training. If someone needed help, she was there. It was common for her to pack a bag and, if she couldn't find transportation, walk twenty or thirty miles to assist. Often she would be gone for several days.

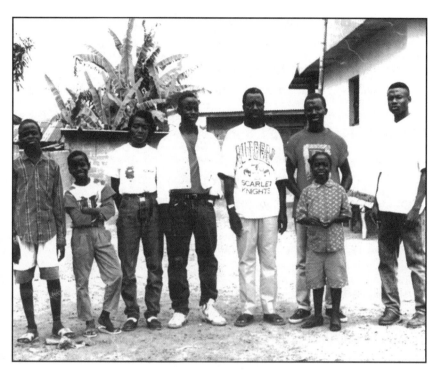

Martha Nehwah's family

"She always gave a helping hand to everybody," says Winnie in her rich voice. "She would try to make friends with you and help you if you needed something. Even with the war going on, she would go out to find relatives and friends and make sure they were still alive. The Wednesday before she died, she set out to find her niece. When she saw that she was well, she went back to Monrovia where she was killed."

Winnie remembers her mother as a stout woman, but she had gotten thinner as the war progressed. Food was harder to come by and she gave much of what she was able to find to her children and grandchildren. She also remembers her mother's unwavering integrity. "She would always advise you to do the right thing," says Winnie. "You didn't ever tell her you did something wrong and ask her to keep it a secret. She would surely tell on you.

"The most important thing my mother taught me was how to be honest and hardworking, how to be nice to people, not just ones you know, but anyone. She taught me how to care for for people."

Florence's selfless service is Winnie's legacy, and Winnie has brought the same spirit not only to her own family, but to Rakhma residents, her church community, and the Liberian community here and in Africa.

There was a funeral for Winnie's mother in Liberia and one in Minneapolis. Without hesitation, relatives and friends, whether they could afford it or not, came from all over the United States to honor Florence at her funeral in Minneapolis. I sat among family, touched by the stories, embraced by the love, included in the circle.

Amara's daughter is eighteen now. She is caught between cultures, having grown up in Cambodia and brought here by her mother who, like Martha, came to make a better life for her children. Amara says her daughter scorns stories of her homeland and wants to forget, adopting instead the trappings of an American teen-ager, including a tendency to rebel against her mother. With relatives still in Cambodia, many dead to the ravages of a savage regime, and with other relatives here, Amara's is a family torn by terror and healed by bonds that cannot be broken by things we Americans only hear about on the news.

Through the quiet heroism demonstrated by so many of the people on Rakhma's staff, Rakhma learns more about what it means to be family, what it means to go the extra mile. Rakhma's diverse staff opens the vista, reminding residents, board members, staff members, family members, and the community alike that the world is small and we are all part of the great, interconnected web of life.

One Affects Many

When the Rakhma Home on Aldrich Avenue South opened, it did not have a name. Several residents were pacers, who all day long walked up and down, back and forth, up the stairs, through the hall, in and out of the kitchen,

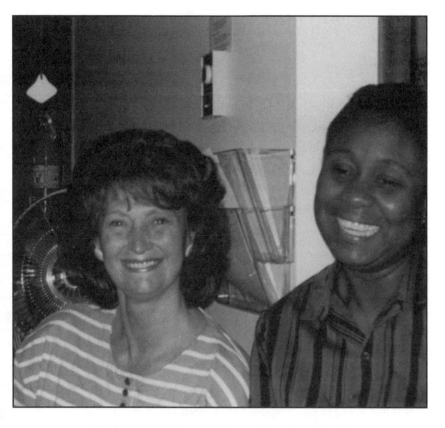

The late Linda Spendel, former house manager,
and Winnie Harris, Rakhma Peace Manager

and through the living room. One day, Seini and I sat down to talk about naming the house. What do we need for this house? As Mary June cruised by, then Helen, then Jean, it was obvious—more peace.

We decided to name it "Peace House." to affirm that peace can exist even in the midst of the residents' agitation.

After a while, we began to look at the larger implications of peace. World peace became a part of daily prayer life. It was decided that this Rakhma home would be a world peace site.

Rakhma Peace Home was dedicated in 1994 to Nelson Mandela, the great South African peacemaker, with this excerpt from his writings a part of the program:

> During my lifetime, I have dedicated myself to this struggle of the African people. I have fought against white domination and I have fought against black domination. I have cherished the ideal of a democratic and free society in which all persons live together in harmony and equal opportunities. It is an ideal which I hope to live for and to achieve. But if need be, it is an ideal for which I am prepared to die.

A five-foot peace pole of carved wood with "May Peace Prevail on Earth" in English, Swahili, Aramaic, and Russian inscribed one on each side, was erected on the corner of the front lawn. The peace pole sprang from The Peace Pole Project, launched in Japan in 1955 by the nondenominational World Peace Prayer Society dedicated to uplift humanity toward harmony rather than conflict. "War begins with thoughts of war...peace with thoughts of peace," says their literature. The peace pole is a reminder to keep peace ever present in our thoughts. To date, friends and supporters have dedicated over one hundred thousand poles in one hundred countries around the world.

Never mind that the week the peace pole was put in, one of the helpers peeked out the front window to discover an older, rather confused woman (not one of our residents) trying to pull it out and bring it home with her. The helper ran out to explain that the pole belonged at Rakhma and that she would have to find one of her own. That afternoon the Rakhma handyman dug a deep hole and anchored the pole with a wheelbarrow full of wet cement

Mr. Mandela received a letter from Rakhma acknowledging him for his great work. Community, family, staff, and residents sat under a striped canopy on a sunny July Sunday, singing songs and sharing thoughts about peace. Full of eats from around the world, everyone left with a clear idea not only about the Rakhma vision of creating a harmonious and peaceful

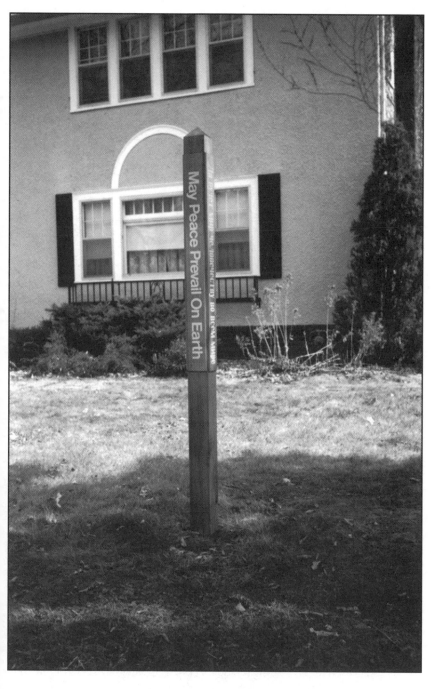

Peace pole at Rakhma Peace Home

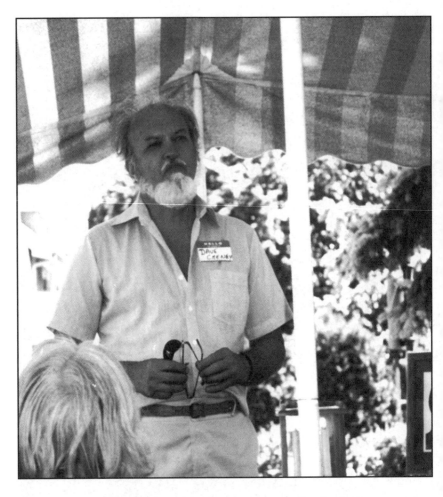

David Cheney at Peace Home dedication

place to live as family, but also having engendered a larger world vision—peace for the entire human family as well.

To Keep in Mind...

- In a shared home setting, residents with dementia have two families—their own children and grandchildren, spouse, siblings, and others involved in their life and care, and residents or staff in the home they may think are their family.

• In a shared home there are sights, sounds, smells, and interactions which stimulate the mind and the senses, keeping residents involved in the workings of the household, and thus living life as normally as is possible.

• A shared home is a nonmedical model. Residents are treated as people who have symptoms, with the emphasis on quality of life. Their disease or symptom is not the primary focus.

• In a shared home the heart of care is the resident.

• More shared homes would make it possible for caregivers to place their loved ones in a noninstitutional setting and get relief from the enormous burden of home care as the loved one's dementia progresses. They would be assured of receiving personal, loving care that emphasizes family involvement.

• The shared home model is small and homelike, yet expands the notion of family to include community.

• The shared home model, by including, supporting and learning from people from all parts of the planet, is an involved member of the the world family.

CHAPTER 4

Finances and Legislation
You Are Not Mother Theresa

Money is more likely to follow the person who has tapped into the
vitality hidden in the things he loves. As we do what we were born
to do, as we love the things we are required to do—even the mundane, even the "dog work"—we stimulate a qualitatively superior
energy within us.
—Marsha Sinetar, *Do What You Love: The Money Will Follow*

The practical clear-sightedness of the people around me was the wind
beneath my visionary wings. Although it felt like those wings were forever being clipped, I knew the pragmatic input of others was the patient
grooming that would allow for healthy growth.

At first the simplest legal questions had to be dealt with. Fresh out of law
school, referred by a friend, Mary Dobbins expressed a long-standing personal
interest in the elderly during our first meeting. She understood the beauty of
the Rakhma vision and the necessity for the kind of care it would make available. Even though there weren't many classes in law school that dealt with
the legal issues of aging, Mary had taken other classes that addressed the social
and personal aspects. My only concern was, should we go profit or nonprofit?
With a nonprofit, could we take care of our helpers? Could we have benefits
for our employees and for myself? Mary said yes, absolutely.

The nurse who was in training to take on major administrative responsibilities at Rakhma did not want to go nonprofit. She envisioned pulling a high

wage with more compensation for her efforts as time went on. Although there is nothing wrong with those aspirations, I was glad to find out in the beginning how differently my nurse and I saw things. I saw the nonprofit as the perfect vehicle for the vision of service with a heart and the philosophy of unconditional love. Where the focus is service, a nonprofit makes sense, and being tax exempt has its advantages when shopping for the needs of the home.

The second time I went to see Mary, the by-laws and articles of incorporation were ready. Of course, with a corporation, I had to have a board. The articles called for five to eight members.

The only thing Mary ever charged for was preparing the articles of incorporation and the by-laws. She somehow got what I was trying to do. Right from the beginning, she encouraged me. She always looked at the bigger picture. Mary has been a steadfast volunteer, another of Rakhma's angels. Still today, fourteen years later, she reads over any Rakhma documents that may have legal ramifications and lends her advice on legal questions.

The Board of Directors

Lynn did a lot of research on nonprofit boards and how to use them. The thing she heard over and over again from executive directors of other nonprofits was, find people who are committed to your vision and who are well connected in the community. Board members are important fund-raisers. Many are willing to serve in that capacity. They are the lifeblood of the non-profit. It made sense to Lynn, since she knew Rakhma had been limping along financially from the beginning. To put it bluntly, Rakhma was in the red.

However, not being financially oriented, I considered Rakhma to be "in the pink." I chose people I admired for my board—a teacher, a retired social worker, a student counselor, a real estate agent. They were friends with no particular interest in fund-raising, but luckily they were financially aware and able to steer the ship aright as time went on.

I felt so rich. All these people who drove a long distance to be at the first meeting and took the time when we only had two residents. It really was happening. We had launched our house and our service. It felt like a wonderful, exciting moment in time.

Original board member Mary Ondov is still on the board. "Shirley doesn't like to think in terms of dollars," she said. "There were times when if it hadn't been for some of the people who loved her concept and loved her, she might have given the store away. We would say in response to one of her ideas, 'That's wonderful but...'

"Shirley knows herself pretty well. The board kept a little hold on her generosity, and Shirley learned. People did it lovingly for the most part, although there were inevitably a few rough spots."

I was looking for people with heart who supported what I was doing. What they could do for the organization financially wasn't a part of it at all. Mary Ondov remembers how, early on, she went to the Littlejohn's Celebration of Life party that is described in Chapter 1. She saw how loving and caring the helpers were with the elderly couple. "Save a spot for me," Mary told me that night. "If I'm going to have to be someplace, I want to be in one of your homes."

Seeing the mission in action deepened her understanding of what I was up to. "It's a service that's alive, loving, full of laughter—a place I would like to be when I get older," Mary said, nodding emphatically.

"Starting that first home was a leap of faith, as I saw it. I became a board member having faith in the concept and in Shirley's belief in it. I saw remarkable things happen. There was never enough money, but she kept giving of her own self and her own money. The stair lift was purely an answer to a prayer. It literally came out of the blue. Being around Shirley I am always reminded, don't lose faith. Shirley has faith. I don't know how it happens, but I go along with it."

In the Red

Even though I still felt "only in the pink," it was clear Rakhma was in the red and losing ground fast. In anticipation of paying off the $104,000 contract for deed, I spoke to my local bank about getting a mortgage. The monthly financial statements weren't looking very good. Although the banker was very kind and encouraged me not to give up, he felt he couldn't risk giving me a mortgage.

The board challenged the wisdom of keeping a person in the home who was being taken care of at one-third the regular fee. I felt I owed a debt of gratitude for being given the opportunity to do this work, and to help care for at least one person who couldn't pay was a way of giving something back.

Fund-raising attempts were begun starting with quick and dirty research about how to do grant writing and where to look for money—from foundations to corporations to individuals. It was an entirely new learning curve, a steep one at that, another plate to spin that needed much more time and attention than I could afford. However, through the blizzard of information and the pile of paperwork needed to solicit and track funding, I got a little snowball rolling with a proposal Lynn wrote up and a fund drive that began with people I knew.

I solicited funds and feedback from everyone I could think of, including my former husband with whom I had corresponded since our 1975 divorce. The relationship remained cordial if a bit formal. He sent regular support payments for the children, and continued sending a monthly sum to me, even after the children were grown.

Jim was living his dream—a position with a prestigious accounting firm in Paris, a mansion on Des Chalet near the Eiffel Tower, a lovely French wife named Nelly who bore him a son. He had it all. Although Jim and I had our differences in the past, I hoped he could separate the Rakhma organization and its vision from his lack of confidence in me.

Rakhma sent Jim a detailed proposal, financial projections, and a request for capital funding. When he declined the proposal, I sent a personal letter requesting that perhaps Jim consider sending the next six months of support payments in advance. His reply, 3 December, 1984:

I was sorry to receive your letter for Thanksgiving where you are asking for the July to December, 1985, payments in advance. The payments will continue as long as I am able, as they have done over all these past years. However, I will not pay it in advance. In any event, it would not be doing you a favor. You may be willing to gamble all on a prayer—not I.

I hope you are receiving qualified advice from your lawyer and that you have entered into this business through a limited liability company arrangement.

Please do not look to me for additional financial aid to what I already provide.... You know that I am already helping our son Jamie.

I regret having to refuse your request but I would only have hoped after all these years that you would be satisfied with what I send and for which you have never had to wait.

I hope it works out for you and that you will in any event have a good Christmas and a very successful 1985.

Affectionately,

Jim

I thanked Jim for his regular monthly sum and gambled all on a prayer as little Rakhma lurched along the bumpy road to self-support.

Not liking to live alone, I rented a room in my lower duplex to my friend Pam Boyce, who later became Rakhma's volunteer coordinator. I loved having Pam in the house and, at the same time, the rent helped offset my mounting expenses. But Pam good-naturedly observed that, since I was never home, I wouldn't know if I had a housemate or not.

I had feelings of real joy. People were living in Rakhma Home whose lives were visibly far better than they had been before. But at night, I would walk straight in from work to the bathtub. After my bath I would lie on the davenport and want to stay there forever. I felt the fatigue that comes with waiting for something to happen, for a turning point.

I refinanced my home and continued to drive my rattly 1976 Ford LTD, later dubbed the Blue Angel by my staff. I didn't draw a salary. After a year and a half, the board implemented a monthly payment schedule of back salary and investment money, to be disbursed along with current salary. Within five years all my accrued salary had been paid plus the money I spent on furnishings and startup.

I was happy to get the money back. I always knew, though, that even if I didn't ever recover my money, it was still worth it. I felt fortunate to be paid back and to start Rakhma. I guess I was a naive investor. Someone told me I fit the entrepreneur profile—love of work, excitement at seeing an idea working, not ever believing it will go down the tubes. But even with a better cash flow there was an undercurrent of anxiety that goes with waiting and waiting and waiting for things to work out financially.

For a short while, I hired helpers as independent contractors, thinking it was okay. The IRS thought differently and demanded a large amount of retroactive employment tax. Plus, paying salaries and payroll taxes before the house was full put a strain on the financial resources. We had a wonderful bookkeeper doing her best to make FICA payments. She'd see what money we had and pay two hundred dollars as a partial payment instead of five hundred dollars full payment. I didn't know you couldn't do that. I thought as long as you paid something, the tax people would understand you were working with them in good faith. The FICA accrued to where the government said, "We've got to have the full payment or we'll come and take all your material goods." I didn't want them taking our residents, too.

Dick Wiessner, a hard-headed businessman who was merely nonplused by my heart-based approach to doing business, was horrified to learn of Rakhma's unique bookkeeping system. Yet he turned out to be another of Rakhma's angels. His heart, too, had been touched as he saw his wife Norma thrive at Rakhma Home, and as he began to feel the joy of life again himself. Dick ensured the continuation of Rakhma by loaning the money to pay off the back FICA and other bills. Then he made corrections in the system, ensuring that a financial black hole would never appear again.

Remember the $104,000 balloon? Well, with a home not quite full, a zoning commission saying that they would only issue a conditional use permit for six people, and all the startup expenses, it was impossible to pay off the contract for deed by 1986. Mr. Helgeson repossessed the house but offered to rent it back to Rakhma. This arrangement bought time, but the rent was increased even though Rakhma paid for major improvements—a fenced-in yard, a finished room in the basement, and a great deal of the building maintenance. The budget remained strained. Even with a full house, the six residents allowed by zoning barely made breakeven.

Almost from the beginning, I had been looking at other houses that might serve as a second shared home. There was a convent for sale, a ten-bedroom colonial home in Minnetonka, a nearby suburb, that was a perfect site for the kind of care Rakhma provides. Ten residents would work financially. We didn't know how we could buy it. I just knew we needed another home. So I began the inquiry that triggered three years of neighborhood and city council meetings addressing concerns about the kind of people a group home would bring into the neighborhood. Mr. Helgeson, who by this time was doing quite well with Rakhma I, became interested in purchasing the convent to rent to the organization.

A Purposeful Investment

By 1988, when the city council and the church board gave Rakhma the go-ahead to buy the convent, Rakhma 1 was running in the black (when it was full) and had proven itself a viable and necessary addition to elder-care options. Mr. Helgeson had already invested his money elsewhere, so where to come up with a down payment was the question of the day. As I went through the process of trying to purchase the convent, I said, "If we buy the home, I want to call it Rakhma Grace Home. It's only by the grace of God we'll be able to buy it!"

Jean Bodine, Grandpa Meili's daughter, came to me and said, "When I was gardening in the backyard, I heard you talking about needing a down payment for a second home. My husband, Cliff, and I have a little savings from the telephone company that we've put away. We could come up with five, maybe even ten thousand dollars."

I couldn't believe my ears. Grandpa Meili was safe and happy in Rakhma I. He wouldn't even be using the second home, yet his daughter was willing to help it come about. She planted a seed in my mind that people from within, friends, would be willing to help. With ten-percent interest on the note, loaning money to Rakhma would be a good investment, but I knew it was more than just a business deal. These investors would be caring people who wanted their money to work for a purpose.

I invited several people to a meeting in my living room. Five people came. There was an informal presentation about Rakhma with slides of the house and the residents. Dick Wiessner helped create a five-year financial projection for the convent, so that when Rakhma approached the bank again for a mortgage, there would be a good, solid financial plan. After some discussion, I asked people to think about what they might be able to invest and passed around a piece of paper torn from a legal pad for pledges. To my amazement, over forty thousand dollars in pledges came in, more than enough for the down payment. I said yes to the full amount, thirty thousand dollars for the down payment, and the rest for work on the new house. Friends of Rakhma, as Rakhma investors are now called, made it possible to buy the convent. This time there was good financial grounding and cash-flow projections that made sense. It's the home that's helped us most. The larger number of residents ensured enough money to operate house number two and helped alleviate problems caused by smaller operating margins at house number one as well. The Friends of Rakhma note was paid off in five years.

The next home, a duplex, was purchased in 1989. A similar community shared-living program in Duluth, Minnesota, found that duplex living worked very well for residents as well as for a smaller organization committed to personal, homelike care. County regulations differ, but in St. Louis County where the Duluth home was located, depending on the bedroom space in the home, you could get an adult foster care license for up to four people and participate in certain Medical Assistance programs. The duplex setting allowed each unit to be licensed separately, making it possible at that time to house up to eight people in the same building and provide excellent centralized care.

In consulting with Tom Patten of the Generations Program in Duluth, I found that Rakhma could make it financially with a duplex. When residents ran out of money, they could be eligible for Medical Assistance, which would cover a portion of their Rakhma costs. People might now be able to stay when their personal funds dwindled, if they wished. This third home, located in a stately St. Paul neighborhood, was also purchased with the help of Friends of Rakhma. Each floor got an adult foster care license. Rakhma Joy Home became a reality.

Around this time, Mr. Helgeson told me he was going to substantially increase the rent at Rakhma Home I. The board suggested I start looking for a duplex in the Minneapolis area that would accommodate eight to ten residents, apply for adult foster care licensing, and move on. I started my search in January 1990, and by August had moved into a spacious gray corner duplex eight blocks away from Rakhma I's original location. It became the first adult foster care home in Hennepin County with shift staffing as opposed to a live-in staff. Shift staffing a shared home was new to the Hennepin County licensing person, but after consulting with the licensing person from Ramsey County who had been working closely with Rakhma in the St. Paul duplex, she was willing to work with it. (See more about shift staffing in Chapter 5.)

Again there were some issues with neighbors, especially the people next door who felt their property value would go down. I assured my new neighbor that my goal was to enhance the property, not let it decline.

Even so, one winter day a resident's grandson pulled into the next door neighbor's driveway to pick up his grandma for chemotherapy, not realizing the driveway did not belong to Rakhma. Incensed, the neighbor complained to authorities and questioned Rakhma's licensing. As is often the case in bureaucratic systems, one hand doesn't know what the other is doing. The licensing department asserted that Rakhma was operating without a license. Of course, with a little checking, they found out we did have a license, but in the meantime, a policewoman came in with a gun on her belt and told me the place would be closed down in five days.

The families of Rakhma residents rallied support by writing to the city council. The councilperson representing the ward in which Rakhma is located consequently found out more about the work Rakhma does and she rallied support. If all else failed, staff members promised to visit me in jail and bring me ice cream. But that's pretty small stuff, someone being in the wrong driveway to pick up his grandmother for chemo. The policewoman had the air of someone who was after the ringleader of a gang. I must admit, we did have our excitement, but all turned out well.

Funding

When Rakhma Joy Home was purchased in Ramsey County, unknown to me, there was a freeze on money for those who could not afford to pay for their care. There was no financial help available from the county or the state and no time line for a thaw. Several residents ran out of money and had to move on.

The licensing people were very pleased we had a home in St. Paul. The adult foster care person knew of our work in Minneapolis and was happy to see Rakhma come across the river. She made special trips to the house and helped us get our first adult foster care license. We did all this thinking we could get Medical Assistance funds.

It was a huge surprise, a huge letdown, when we couldn't, but we didn't allow ourselves to stay in that place for very long. Judy Melinat, my assistant and I, sat on the porch of Joy Home, looked at each other, and said, "We're not going away. We will find another way to do this."

Judy went down to the Medical Assistance offices to look into the situation. Dick Wiessner rattled a few cages in the legislature, and family members of residents met with people to ask why there was a freeze on Medical Assistance funding for an adult foster care home. My mom needs this kind of care, they would say, and we don't want to put her in a nursing home when her personal funds run out.

All our efforts must have made a difference, but at the time we were making them, we were given no indication that anyone in the bureaucracy was listening. Soon, however, Ramsey County sent a letter saying funds were available and that Rakhma was an approved provider. We could now submit the paperwork necessary to receive Medical Assistance funding for residents who had applied and were eligible.

This is one of the problems the home-setting model runs into. At conferences and conventions, other professionals have approached me, frustrated in their attempts to create a similar model. After researching the field, each one of them became discouraged by bureaucratic red tape, lack of adequate Medical Assistance funding, zoning ordinances, and a myriad of hoops that give a small home with a small staff and a small budget great headaches.

I wouldn't recommend it—too many headaches—but this is where a ready, fire, aim style of operating made a difference. I saw myself caring for elderly people, so I bought a house and just did my work. The red tape I encountered was on-the-job training in hoop jumping; much staff time is still spent in meetings learning how the legislature works, how the city works, how foster care and regulatory bodies work. Rakhma is very small among the giants of the system, but it is a voice that must be heard. I intend that my experience forge the way for others to make personalized care available and affordable nationwide. Each city, county, and state has different rules, regulations, and disbursement of monies. It is my intention that shared homes leave the realm of alternative housing forever and become as much a part of our elder-care system as nursing homes are now, allowing those who choose a smaller setting to remain eligible for the same funding they would get in a larger setting.

After the initial application, it was more than a year and a half before the first Medical Assistance check came in, not the couple of months I thought it would take to get the system in place. Some residents who had run out of private pay money were now eligible for partial Medical Assistance coverage in the home setting. Their families were relieved that their loved ones would be able to stay. Rakhma kept operating on the promise of reimbursement with no reimbursement coming forth.

A few residents left because of the financial hardship and uncertainty. The board was ready to have us let go entirely. They were really frustrated. After all the headaches, they wanted us to be private pay only and not deal with Medical Assistance at all, but, of course, that leaves so many people out.

During that hard time, I felt as if I was a ship out on the water alone. When we got a check in the mail for forty-two thousand dollars, it was a last minute save. I made a copy of the check and passed it around at the board meeting. I thought the board would be much more excited than they were, but I think they had almost given up! We still have a funny stuffed doll propped in the office with a tag I hung on her that says "$42,000 arrived May 2, 1992!" I look with awe at the saving grace of how, when there have been difficult times, what we need comes forth.

The Medical Assistance battle tempered my vision of having room for those who couldn't pay with the practical considerations of having enough cash flow to keep the doors open. I knew Rakhma had to be careful about how much public funding it accepted, so if money didn't come in the houses wouldn't go under. Although I would like Medical Assistance to be available for at least fifty percent of our residents, for such a small organization the board has limited assisted funding to twenty-five percent, with seventy-five percent of fees to remain private pay.

Optimum Size

The first house, Rakhma Home I, was licensed as a board and lodging facility for eight people, pending zoning approval. Zoning wouldn't hear of having eight unrelated people in a residential neighborhood, but with the care program already in place, and a good one at that, the zoning people weren't quite sure what to do with Rakhma. Someone on the zoning board understood what the home was about and wrote a proposal for a new zoning category—Special Home Care for the Elderly. In the end, Rakhma was allowed to stay, but was given a conditional use permit for only six people that had to be renewed every year. It soon became apparent that at least seven full-pay people were needed to carry the expenses. The board discussed options and decided that a second home would help defray the huge overhead that one small home demanded.

The second home, as mentioned before, was a stately colonial that had previously been a convent built for the nuns who taught at the Immaculate Heart of Mary School. The large comfortable living room, spacious kitchen, and recreation room in the basement gave it a homey feeling, while at the same time it had many bathrooms with two private stalls in each to accommodate more than one person at a time, one bathroom with three sinks, and ten bedrooms, some with their own sinks. It was perfect.

The cash flow from that home helped run the first home. Named Rakhma Grace, it was the saving grace in the early years because it always ran in the black. Through trial by fire, Rakhma has found that between nine to ten residents per house allows for individualized care to work financially.

A New Paradigm: Consumer-Driven Care

You can't license a shared home like an institution. So often institutional regulations, though meant to benefit the health and safety of the resident, are too narrow. The individual gets lost. Results of consumer surveys are now bearing out what we pioneered.

The number one finding in the 1990 Seniors Agenda for Independent Living Report is that seniors do not want to be institutionalized. Seniors want to be given options as to where they live and how they are cared for if they become frail. The problem with current nursing home regulations in most states is that, although designed to protect the resident, they do so by imposing strict cut-and-dried standards. An inspector comes in, surveys the establishment, checks off a compliance list, orders the rug off the floor in a resident's room or nonporous upholstery for all furniture. The place ticks like clockwork, the resident is relatively safe, all surfaces are shiny, and anything that is deemed a risk to life or limb has been removed from the premises. However, a sense of home has also been removed, and though clean and virtually risk-free, the elderly person's life is no longer their own.

We want homes where people can help with the cooking, where they can be involved. We feel very strongly that the rules should be flexible enough to allow us to respond to the consumer. What are their needs when they come in? What are their needs as they change while they are with us? It makes sense that the consumer can make requests, ask how the home can provide this or that, instead of us telling people, "This is only what this house does, this is only what the state allows."

Nursing homes are locked into a giant array of regulations, says John Kitto, former Executive Director of the Alzheimer's Association of Minnesota. Even though there are visionaries within the nursing-home industry, making changes in the system and proposing new approaches to care, life in a nursing home is structured around caring for physical needs only. Management responds to the marketplace and to regulatory bodies in a very bureaucratic environment.

"Then, it's not a home anymore," says Kitto. "The spark has gone away. Home is supposed to serve. Someone with Alzheimer's disease needs technical help, of course, but most of all they need a warm, special place."

In a small place like Rakhma, one can go back to providing a home. What makes Mary or Joe happy? A decision can be made in the morning and by noon it can take place. In nursing homes such flexibility is hard and complex.

"To a person with Alzheimer's, community and continuity are important," says Kitto. "When you go to live with a huge number of people, that gets lost. Lifestyle and community are disrupted.

"Just stand at end of a nursing home hall and look down it. People don't live like that, except when they're in a college dorm. You can't link with others. A smaller group aesthetic allows for community. I don't see the nursing home industry embracing this. The opportunity to live in a homelike environment is almost nonexistent, at least here in the upper Midwest.

"When I go to Rakhma, Shirley doesn't show me the new computer system with the latest software or the new paint color. She doesn't worry about whether the pattern on the drapes is too busy. The first thing she does is introduce me to the people who live there. It's their home. That's normality in life. She deals with how people want to live, how they would want to be in their home.

"Momentarily I think, oh my God, this isn't as safe as it should be. Is this going to fit the regulations? But the normality, the care, the love is what I really see and wish I saw it at more facilities. In the debate between facts and figures versus having coffee and watching the birdies in the morning, watching the birdies is what it's all about."

He says there is a need for financial restructuring in elder care as well as a need for spiritual awakening. Minnesota is addressing some of these issues.

As frail older people increasingly live in community settings rather than nursing homes, state officials have examined the need for additional regulation of these settings. A major concern has been that nursing-home type regulations would force residential settings to become more institutional, clearly contrary to consumer preferences. Beginning in 1993 the Minnesota Association of Homes for the Aging—now the Minnesota Health &

Housing Alliance (MHHA)—began examining various other ways of promoting quality care in housing-with-service settings, which is what Rakhma and many smaller care providers are. A number of quality assurance options were examined during numerous meetings with providers, five consumer focus groups, advocacy groups, and state officials. Out of this a new regulatory model has been developed that contains three very basic conceptual changes:

1. Centrality of the consumer (resident). Consumers and providers in MHHA's meetings have emphasized that the welfare and quality of life of the consumer (resident) are inseparable from the consumer' ability to exercise choice and maintain autonomy. In the current long-term care system, the welfare of the resident is the goal, yet the system developed to meet that goal has often been directed by someone other than the resident. Although providers, consumers, and regulators have all become accustomed to that pattern, the result has been institutionalized settings that consumers want to avoid.

2. Risk. A system that demands and supports the primacy of the consumer calls for a change in the way risk is considered. A system based on choice cannot have the elimination of risk as its goal. Rather, such a system must seek to manage the risk that is inherent with any real exercise of choice.

3. Standardization versus customer satisfaction. In long-term care, consumers, providers, and regulators have become accustomed to a system in which standards are clear, measurable, and universal, resulting in standardized services. In a system that relies on individual choices, the focus shifts from a standardized measurement of service delivery to a concern for the supports necessary to assure informed and competent decision making. The final test in such a system is customer satisfaction rather than performance according to prescribed procedures.

Consumer-driven regulation would be brought about by shifting to a contract model. In other words, establishments would enter into contracts with residents or residents' representatives, should, as with Alzheimer's disease, the residents be unable represent themselves. These contracts would be subject to statutory requirements regarding the execution and contents of contracts. This sort of regulation assures elder care that is not driven by the reimbursement mechanism, but instead is driven more directly by the wishes of the individual consumer.

MHHA has developed the Elderly Housing with Services Contract Act, which was passed by the 1995 Minnesota legislature. (A year later, to be more inclusive, the title was changed to Housing with Services.) Under this act, a contract between the housing-with-services provider and the senior resident serves as the primary mechanism for assuring customer satisfaction and quality services in these settings. In addition, the establishments covered by the act must register with the Department of Health, which has standing to petition the court should the establishment not fulfill the terms of the contract or fail to comply with other applicable laws. The act also requires home-care licensure in settings that provide health-related services.

The Licensing Soup

Rakhma Grace, the former convent, is currently considered a board and lodging facility registered with the city of Minnetonka to provide services, a category originated for hotels that has never been changed. The number of people allowed in a board and lodge is restricted by the physical size of the facility and certain zoning requirements (e.g., special use permit). Originally, ten was the maximum number of residents allowed by the licensure of the Minnetonka home, but in 1993 I applied for permission to fill an eleventh room with one more resident, and to my delight the request was granted. The other two homes, because they are duplexes and house no more than five people per unit, are adult foster care homes. (The ruling for the number of people allowed per unit changed from four to five after the duplexes were originally licensed.)

There are now Elderly Waiver funds that provide Medical Assistance money for care to people more than sixty years old. The hitch is that if anyone else in the unit is under sixty, and this is sometimes the case with the early onset of Alzheimer's disease, no one there can receive Elderly Waiver funding.

The adult foster care law was evolved to address the special needs of dependent adults in a home setting and to prevent abuse and neglect of vulnerable adults. In an adult foster care home, there is a semiannual visit from a county social worker who walks through the house, visits with each resident, reviews their records, and reviews personnel information. I feel the adult foster care rules are quite flexible, giving the home leeway to provide individualized care. Medical Assistance programs, however, do not cover all aspects of the care and services provided in residential care facilities. Less money is reimbursed in the home setting than in the nursing-home setting.

A nursing home has a licensed professional on duty twenty-four hours a day. Although there are relatively few caregivers in proportion to the number of residents in a nursing home, especially at night, regulatory bodies are in the habit of looking for credentials first as a criteria for funding. Rakhma offers the same nonmedical services as a nursing home does, but with *much more personal attention available to residents twenty-four hours a day.* Along with the caregivers on duty in each of the homes, there is a registered nurse on call at all times, as well as myself, my co-director Judy Cline (who came on board in 1995) or another qualified administrator. The absence of a round-the-clock licensed professional is one thing that limits the amount of public reimbursement monies available.

Another thing is that in a nursing home, housing and services are considered to be a whole highly regulated package, and the cost of housing and its regulation is wrapped into fee for services. In a home like Rakhma, housing and services are considered separate. Therefore, reimbursement for services does not include cost of housing, which, of course, is essential to serving the Alzheimer's resident. Housing and services in a shared home model go hand in glove, but this is not taken into account by government programs.

For these reasons, anybody who is getting reimbursement in our homes is getting that much less than it costs to provide care in our homes. In many cases, family members pay the fee differential.

There are people who feel that fees and services should be standardized. However, standardized care undermines the ability of the facility to customize care and respond to change.

At this time, the idea of a standard fee for adult foster care services is being kicked around the regulatory meetings in the state of Minnesota, an idea that Rakhma strongly opposes. That approach standardizes care to the lowest common denominator, and a small home with more overhead per person cannot maintain itself. It spells out fairly narrow parameters regarding the kinds of services a home setting can provide, and makes it necessary for people to move to other settings as they become frailer. It doesn't take into account that residents who choose a home setting like Rakhma intend to live out their lives there. Of course, sometimes frail residents get to a point of needing more medical care than Rakhma is equipped to provide, in which case they would go to a hospital or nursing home. However, many elderly people simply become frailer, needing more nonmedical care as time goes on, and could stay in a shared home with the help of caring, nonmedical staff until their death. The problem with standard fee for services is that when a person enters an adult foster care facility, they become locked in to a set fee, which doesn't take into account a variety of levels of care. This set fee is required to be less expensive than the cost of a nursing home. In a nursing home there are many levels of care and fee structures to reflect overhead more accurately.

We're talking about people living their lives out in homes like ours. Even though it's not a medical setting, care needs will change. People need more assistance, more attention from staff as their ability to help themselves decreases. A standard fee rule would mean getting $1,000 to $1,500 less than it costs for people who need a lot of care. We couldn't provide the quality that they came here for in the first place. We're looking at men and women with dementia, not independent people who need supervision and nothing else.

This presents a quandary. Even though, in theory, fees in Minnesota are based on services right now, the ideal for customized care, services are limited by a cap. The result is very much like a standard fee anyway because there is only so much a person can receive as a result of the reimbursement system for our kind of setting.

With the exception of the nuclear industry, nursing homes are the most highly regulated industry in the country. With regulation comes money for reimbursement, and with money comes regulation. This is another quandary we have not been able to resolve. Perhaps as more people become aware of the viability of community shared homes such as Rakhma, legislation will support their existence, making it possible to offer fitting choices to those who do not need a medical model and who prefer a homelike setting.

Everything is up for discussion right now in Minnesota. A new set of rules is in the making, but we don't know where things will fall when it comes to reimbursement. As Judy Cline says, "All we can do right now is jump in, stay aware and awake, and swim."

We have people like little Isabel who couldn't walk at all the last three years of her life here, or eat by herself, yet she lived here among friends until she died. I can't see why people have to leave because they need more care, especially when we're assessing day to day, week to week. I feel they should be able to die here in their home, with their own pictures on wall, and not have to be rushed off to a nursing home at their time of dying because we can't afford to keep them or they don't fit into a neat category.

Changes in Paris

At fifty-five, my former husband, Jim, retired as partner in charge of the Paris office of Peat, Marwick & Mitchell after a traumatic merger accompanied by a lot of stress. After retirement, he and Nelly began to notice problems with his memory. As his forgetfulness increased, he was astounded that he could no longer find words for simple, everyday objects like "dog" or "bicycle," but he would laugh it off, making jokes about aging as if he weren't at all worried. The future he had so single-mindedly worked for was his. He had caught the brass ring, and nothing was going to mar the accomplishment.

I noticed it in letters. Jim had always prided himself on his precise spelling and proper English grammar. Now he misspelled things and his sentence structure began to deteriorate.

The year we opened our third shared home for people with Alzheimer's disease, Jim came to the United States for daughter Liz's wedding. As Jim hobnobbed with family and friends, I observed the extent of his memory loss and was taken aback by its severity. I suggested to Nelly it would be a good thing for Jim to have a neurological exam. Neither Nelly nor Jim wanted to know if anything was really wrong.

"He won't go to a doctor," Nelly announced. "I've talked with him about it before."

How to approach this? How to do what must be done? Now I faced the question that family members of our residents and prospective residents face every day.

Talking with Jim on the phone after he returned to Paris, I urged him to have an exam—if not for himself, for Nelly. "If there is something wrong, she will need to know. Working with people with Alzheimer's disease, I know that sometimes early diagnosis can make a difference. Maybe you could work with it for a while."

A few months later, in the fall of 1990, I made an appointment for Jim at the Neurology Clinic at the University of of Minnesota. As Nelly does not like to fly, Jim traveled by himself and stayed at my place. Dr. David Knopman examined him.

The day of the exam, Jim had a temper tantrum. "I'm not going," he shouted as we were ready to leave for the clinic. I tried to keep cool. This,

I knew, was something Jim was afraid of doing. He didn't want to know. He didn't want to shatter his hopes for the future. He consented to go only with the promise of tea afterward at Dick Wiessner's in St. Paul.

Everything went wrong when we got to Dr. Knopman's office. Jim was cross about needing his social security number; he didn't want to cooperate with people in the records department. He strode about the office, agitated, rude, and angry.

However, when he met with Dr. Knopman, he became talkative and quite clear. He told Dr. Knopman about doing important work in Paris, how he was a respected man with much responsibility. "Now, though, something is wrong with my head and I can't remember anything."

Knowing he had a doctor to listen to him, he poured his heart out. I sat right there with him.

"I don't know anything about food anymore. I can't remember the names of things I'm eating."

"Can you name those?" Dr. Knopman said, pointing to Jim's fingers.

"No."

"What is this?" Dr. Knopman touched Jim's knee.

"I don't know."

They went through all the body parts, one by one. Jim could not remember.

"Doctor, I'm concerned." Jim pointed to his groin area. "The thing down there hasn't worked in three years. I have a beautiful wife. It bothers me; it worries me that it doesn't work anymore."

Dr. Knopman listened. He asked about Paris and how the plane ride had gone.

I held back tears. Love doesn't die. Mine wasn't the kind of love that still wanted to be married to Jim. It was the love that cuts to the heart of the situation, that recognizes the essence of a person and responds despite difficulty, distance, and fundamental philosophical differences. This was my children's father, a man who now needed the kind of expertise and resources I could provide.

After his appointment with Dr. Knopman, Jim went on for further tests at the university clinic, where he worked with shapes and tried to answer more questions. I stayed nearby. After it was all over I dropped Jim off at Dick's for tea and cookies and went to join a tour of Rakhma Joy Home. I found the group upstairs, almost finished with the tour, pleased to see such workable alternative housing in their community. I thanked everyone for coming, and without planning to, shared what I had just been through with Jim. "I realize more deeply than ever what family members go through, the courage you have and the terrible sadness you feel," I said through stinging tears.

Jim flew back to Paris and Nelly. Dr. Knopman prepared a report to send to Jim's physician in Paris with a copy to me:

Dear Doctor Hewes:

At the request of Mr. Shaw's ex-wife, with whom he was visiting in Minneapolis, I had occasion to see Mr Shaw on October 22 in the Alzheimer's Disease and Memory Disorders Clinic at the University of Minnesota. According to notes supplied by the patient's current wife who lives with him in Paris, as well as reports from the patient, Mr. Shaw has experienced significant difficulties with word finding and forgetfulness over at least the past three years.

We obtained psychometric testing on Mr. Shaw and it confirmed that he had a fairly dense amnesic disorder. In addition, he had significant problems with language function in that his word fluency and his naming were extremely poor. On the other hand, his nonverbal reasoning abilities were largely preserved. Thus, Mr. Shaw appears to have a dementing illness that would be compatible with Alzheimer's disease.

Dr. Knopman recommended Jim get support in Paris and that his wife should be aware that he could get worse in one to three years. Nelly was given this diagnosis by Dr. Hewes, but she didn't believe it. After two more specialists in Paris confirmed the diagnosis, she realized that life was not going to be the same. For a while, Jim took some trial medication that the doctors recommended, but Nelly saw no difference in his functioning, so she took him off it.

Jim's last visit to the states was in 1991. In the spring of '92, my friend Pam and I visited Jim in Paris. Together we explored churches, enjoyed dinner at good restaurants, took leisurely walks down tree-lined streets. Jim was his old difficult self most of the time. He was rude to Nelly and to Mark, his son.

"You are so lucky to have Nelly in your life," I reminded him. "She is such a wonderful wife." Jim put one arm around me and one around Nelly. "What is your name? Shirley Joy Shaw. What is your name? Nelly Shaw. And my name is Shaw. So see. We are all related."

Nelly said "Yes. He's got a harem." And everyone laughed.

In his disease Jim had become increasingly irritable and self-centered. My four children and I remember him that way from the early years. Married about fifteen years before the onset of Alzheimer's, Nelly says she's had very good years with Jim. "If he was that way before," asked Nelly, "how could you stand it?"

After I left the marriage, Jim had some time to reflect. In a letter, he wrote, "I am very remorseful of not making time for you and the children." He soon met Nelly, made changes, worked shorter hours, arranged to spend more weekend time at home. Throughout the marriage, Jim brought Nelly fresh flowers every Friday after work. His efforts gave them the good years.

Jim can no longer write letters. The last one he sent, however, was different from the rest:

April 1, 1993
Dear Shirley,
It was nice our speaking. And I hope you are always in good shape.
I am sending you the support again and for April, May, June.

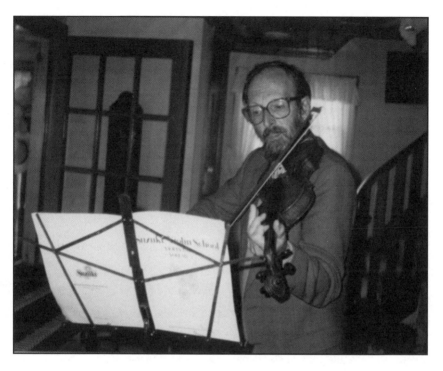

Jim Shaw playing during his last visit to Minnesota

We had been thinking that you were to come over to Paris and we could do things to take care of you. But you said now that you are not coming over. I hope you are happy.

Nelly thinks of you and she would like to see you regularly.

It is nice to talk to you.

We love you Shirley.

James and Nelly

I love you Shirley—James—I love you.

As Jim declined, he could still play piano but not the violin. A companion took him for walks every day and Nelly did the rest. The days were down to a routine—two baths, a walk, meals. After his mother died, he would sit in the bathtub repeating "Mother…Shirley…God…" over and over again.

When Becky and Liz, two of our daughters, visited their father in Paris in March1994, he didn't recognize them as his children. Nelly had chosen a facility for him for when she could no longer care for him, but she wanted to keep him home as long as possible.

As time went by, Jim got more and more compulsive. He wanted to go for walks all the time. When on a walk, he would run away from Nelly, out into the busy street, arms up as if he were God stopping traffic. In April 1995, Jim entered a small Paris facility for twelve people that specializes in Alzheimer's disease and is owned by a doctor.

Although he thought all the women on the staff there were delicious, adjustment was extremely hard for Jim. He resisted taking off his clothes for days. Nelly did not visit again until he got acclimated.

If Jim were here in America, maybe he'd be in a Rakhma Home. Before his illness, he had no time for the homes, either as a financial contributor or as a visitor when he stayed with me on his trips to America. The residents were not neat and orderly as he liked. Their behavior was too random. They were unrefined. After his illness progressed, however, he enjoyed the Rakhma homes. They were wonderful and beautiful, homelike and charming. He would talk to people, he saying this, they saying that, and he didn't care that the conversations were disjointed. He played his violin for the appreciative residents.

He received the quarterly Rakhma newsletters in Paris and he tried to read and understand them. He felt an affinity now. One day he said, "Shirley, you've accomplished so much. You've done so much. I'm so proud of you that you're doing this housing for people."

I have taken this acknowledgement as the greatest gift. I understand that the money Jim did send, although it could be considered alimony, was really a gift to me from him. It was what he could see to do at the time before he understood the scope of our work. His support was an important part of Rakhma happening, a financial resource that allowed us to keep going in the face of many months of no income.

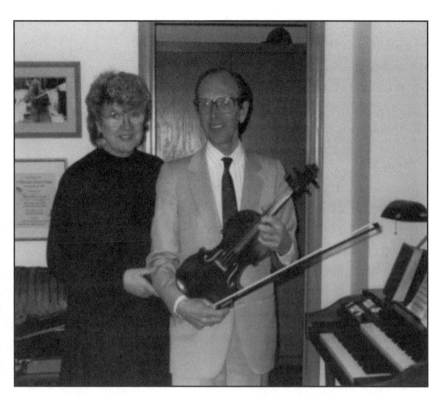

Shirley Shaw and Jim Shaw at Rakhma Grace Home

I would like to go to Paris again to see Jim once more. Maybe he'll recognize me, maybe not. I'd like to walk with him and see the home he lives
in. I want to give him one last hug.

David Whyte, in his poem "Self Portrait," responds to this puzzle of
what's here to do, what drives this desire to serve. His words reach into the
corners of my life as if he knew my story. Rather, I think, mine is the human
story of being drawn into life by one's commitments, of being moved by
one's vision so powerfully that one goes beyond the mundane into the spiritual. Whyte says:

...I want to know if you are prepared to live in the world
with its harsh need
to change you. If you can look back
with firm eyes
saying this is where I stand. I want to know
if you know
how to melt into the fierce heat of living
falling toward
the center of your longing. I want to know
if you are willing
to live, day by day, with the consequence of love
and the bitter
unwanted passion of your sure defeat.

I have been told, in *that* fierce embrace, even
the gods speak of God.

To Keep in Mind...

- For a model like Rakhma to work, the commitment must come from the heart, not the pocketbook.

- There are people who have both a heartfelt commitment to loving homelike care and who are financially astute, willing to invest in, advise, and lend assistance to a shared-home model that is not money driven. These are the kind of people you want to invite to work with you as vision becomes reality.

- Don't lose faith, even when there are seemingly insurmountable obstacles.

- Caring investors want their money to work for a purpose. A sound model like Rakhma's provides a return on investment and an opportunity to contribute to the greater good.

- Be aware that when working with public funding there is a great deal of bureaucratic red tape. Public funding can be unreliable, unpredictable, and subject to change.

- Consumer-driven care is the new paradigm in elder care. It ensures quality of life based on choice and managed risk. It allows the resident or resident's representative to work out a contract with a nonmedical facility that is personalized, dignified, and flexible. In Minnesota, the Housing with Services Contract Act creates a framework for this kind of care.

- At this time there are still funding problems regarding care for people who have become more frail, do not need medical care, and wish to age in place. Current funding guidelines do not include a category for the extra nonmedical care a frail person requires. When a home like Rakhma can no longer be reimbursed for the level of care required, the only alternative is to send the resident to a nursing home.

- Always there is a bigger picture. This is a human story. We are shifting our consciousness to understand what it means to care for people with dignity and love. It can be done from a heartfelt commitment that includes fiscal viability but does not put profit before people.

CHAPTER 5

Making Changes

You can't help respecting anybody who can spell TUESDAY, even if he doesn't spell it right; but spelling isn't everything. There are days when spelling Tuesday simply doesn't count.

—Benjamin Hoff, *The Tao of Pooh*

As people become more confused, change can be hard. There comes a time when they can't express themselves, so they may get angry or act out in some way. In the early stages of memory loss, people know they are going through changes but can't verbalize it.

There isn't any predictable length of time that the first stage lasts because people deal with it in different ways. Often years go by before memory loss becomes identifiable to others. A person may have to work much harder in their thinking process to continue a job, or they may keep copious notes to maintain a normal social schedule, but they can usually cover lapses quite well for a while. There comes a time, though, when there has been enough change that others are affected.

Muriel, punctual as high noon, didn't show up for her hair appointment three weeks in a row. Her hairdresser was miffed, phoned, then realized Muriel was not tracking very well. Rob's mom, a woman who loves to send a funny card, forgot his birthday. Even in middle age, Rob felt slightly orphaned. He could always rely on his mom and now she'd forgotten him. It woke him up, however, to other small incidents, and he realized something had changed. These sorts of scenarios gather momentum, the little lapses coming closer and closer together until they can no longer be concealed or denied. A family member finds that, over time, they have become a caregiver. As the disease progresses, more and more is required of the caregiver until he or she reaches the point of needing outside help. This part of the Alzheimer's disease process is detailed in Chapter 3, with the story of Dick Wiessner and his wife Norma.

Changes continue, of course, all along the way. This chapter addresses some of the things that occur in the intermediate stages of the disease, during the time when a person is being cared for in a Rakhma home and up to the time when they must leave because they need more medical care. The following story is typical of the kinds of changes that a person with Alzheimer's disease may go through. It shows how change can be sudden from one day to the next, making it essential that caregivers and family respond appropriately, and it underscores the kinds of ongoing decisions that must be made as behavior and needs change, keeping in mind the dignity of the resident and others involved.

Louis was a slim, wiry man with deep brown eyes like a water spaniel's. His career as an engineer took him to countries all over the world, where he managed large projects and many people. He was a "take charge" kind of guy.

Both in their eighties, Louis and his wife, Catherine, had lived all fifty-eight years of their married life in Indiana. In 1983, Louis was diagnosed with Alzheimer's disease. Catherine thought she could cope with it, despite Louis's occasional outbursts of aggressive behavior. One night when she blocked him from leaving the house with his suitcases, he tried to choke her, convinced she was a man keeping him from leaving for work. After that, Louis went into the hospital for observation and behavior management medication. A few months later, Catherine suffered a severe stroke and was not expected to live.

Louis's son, Philip, who lives in Minneapolis, placed him in Rakhma Home I hoping it would be easier there for him to adjust to all the change he was going through. The staff was pleased to have Louis as a resident. He brought a smile to Gerry's face, the youngest resident, who, at fifty-seven,

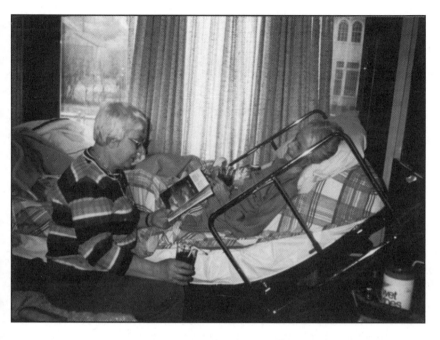

Catherine enjoying Vi Banks, a volunteer
friend from Judson Memorial Baptist Church

had severe Alzheimer's symptoms. Louis would watch her and say, "I love you, Judy," over and over every day. To him, Gerry was Judy, his handicapped daughter who had lived at home with her parents until her death a few years earlier. Louis became Gerry's protector. Although he soon became annoyingly overprotective, having "Judy" around kept him happy for a while.

Louis became increasingly more difficult. He fancied himself as overseer of the household, and every day sat in the same spot on the sofa in the living room directing activity.

When Catherine had recovered enough to be moved, the family asked if Rakhma would be willing to have her in the home with Louis. She was frail from the stroke and needed a lot of assistance, but her mind was sharp. The staff knew they would be taking on a great deal of additional care with Catherine in the home, but they also considered the possibility that

Louis would be happier and perhaps more manageable, that she might provide him with a link to reality. Another plus was keeping a couple together, a vision that I maintained ever since working with the Littlejohns in the very beginning.

Catherine arrived on a cold, rainy October day after a long ride in a private plane from her Indiana hospital bed. When she was lifted out of the car into the wheelchair and pushed along the sidewalk to the front door, Louis, the staff, and I lined up in the front hallway, waiting in eager anticipation. I said, "Louis, look who's coming!"

When he saw her, his eyes lit up. "She's mine!" he crowed. After four months of being apart, they embraced, hugged, kissed, and cried. There wasn't a dry eye in the crowd.

Later, after Catherine was settled in her bed, Louis's grandson and I brought him upstairs to see her. For Louis, it was like seeing her for the first time again. He went down on his knees, embracing her and crying. "I love you, Catherine. I love you." Said the grandson, "I think this is the greatest love story on earth."

Though Louis was delighted to be with Catherine at first, his Alzheimer's disease progressed rapidly. He had lost twenty pounds, which made him physically frailer, yet he became more aggressive. After about a month, he spent less time with her, telling her he had things to do, and he would go off and disturb the peace of others in the house. Catherine was having her own difficulties coping with the aftermath of a stroke.

She could no longer use her right hand or leg and was unable to walk. Speaking was extremely difficult. She had said good-bye to lifelong friends in Indiana. She wanted to go home and knew she couldn't. She needed to be near her son and grandsons who lived in Minnesota. It was a depressing situation and her husband's disinterest made her sadder.

One day when the residents were gathered in the living room listening to Bob, a staff member, play the piano, Louis noticed ninety-two-year-old Ernest slouched back on the couch snoring with his mouth wide open. He rushed at Ernest, declaring, "I don't want a lazy man sleeping on the job." When I placed myself between Ernest and Louis, Louis threatened to knock my block off. He was out of control.

Catherine, who rarely spoke plainly, screamed, "I want him to go!" Taken aback, I asked, "Are you saying you want your husband to go?"

"Yes," she screamed.

"Where do you want him to go?" I asked in shock.

In tears, Catherine murmured, "I don't care."

Louis had moved in to Rakhma in June 1986. Catherine joined him in October. In March 1987, Louis was placed in a nursing home. The cost of keeping Louis was too high; his behavior affected the other residents, staff, family members, volunteers, and even Honey, the house dog. Keeping Catherine and Louis together as a couple became unrealistic.

Louis's departure brought peace again to Rakhma. Catherine began getting up to eat at the dining-room table and occasionally went on outings to Lake Harriet in her wheelchair with the others. She made new friends and seemed happier, though she missed Louis. When he was brought to visit her for a coffee party every week, her eyes would light up. She would gaze at him lovingly, straighten his shirt collar, pat his hand. Though he always seemed happy to see Catherine, he was oblivious to her concerns and didn't seem to miss her when he was away. After his last sip of coffee, he would put on his hat and be ready to go. Every time after he left, Catherine would cry bitter, silent tears, so bonded in her love yet so alone in her grief.

In the meantime, I visited Louis regularly in the nursing home, often accompanied by staff member Susie and her mandolin. He seemed to be on good behavior, leaving the other residents to themselves, perhaps thinking he was in a hotel. Anything is possible in the Alzheimer's world.

Although it no longer fit for Catherine to be with Louis, he was always in her heart and on her mind. She knew even as she and Louis became too frail to visit each other that I would make the visits, come back, and tell her truthfully just how Louis was.

Human behavior is complex, and the decisions that are called for as the person with Alzheimer's disease changes are not always easy. Louis went through many stages, from somewhat functional with some aggression to highly aggressive and unmanageable.

The process demands great attention from caregivers and family members, not only to the individual's changing needs but also to the needs of others in the household. Some people remain stable for years at a time and do not change as quickly as Louis did. Others change even more quickly and must be moved to a more appropriate environment for their medical or behavioral needs. Some people with memory loss move into a more peaceful, less agitated state as time goes by. Some stay to die at Rakhma in a loving, hospice-like environment. More will follow on the continuum of care through death in Chapter 9.

Gently Changing

When there's an opening in one of the homes, thinking ahead about changes makes it possible to implement the changes gently. Staff members give a lot of thought to who may need to move to a different room and how much time they may need to do it. The key question is, "What are the current residents' needs?" If there is a first-floor opening, it might be time to move a frailer person from upstairs to that first-floor room. When a new person moves into a double room, there is a trial period to help each person acclimate. Moving the beds in a familiar configuration often helps a person with Alzheimer's disease to adjust more easily to new surroundings.

Alice did fine the first night she was in her new room, but the next night woke up in the wee hours of the morning and headed back to her old room, which of course was occupied now by someone else. Being that she was an early riser anyway, staff invited her to have toast and juice in those early mornings when she would get anxious, and soon she settled more peacefully into her new space.

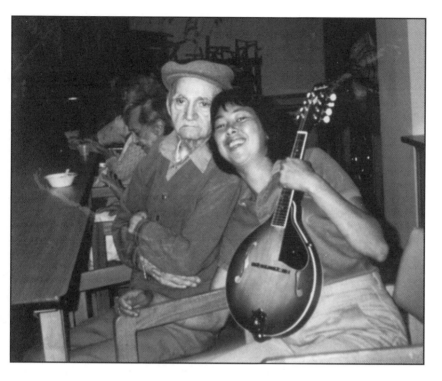

Louis with Susie Gilbert bringing music to the nursing home

When we have new people coming in and sharing a room with some-one, it can be very stressful. It depends on how advanced they are in their dementia. If they have a kind nature and advanced dementia, sharing is easier. They may rummage through the other person's clothes a bit and take several days to settle down, but they will likely get along okay. Some peo-ple are very territorial, and get more so as their disease advances. They defend their space, mostly through acting out or aggressive behavior.

Marcella came in having been on heavy medication in a nursing home. She sat, staring, in a chair in the living room the first week she was at Rakhma, unresponsive to her surroundings until the medication was out of her system. We would rather have her with her personality intact than as a zombie. Her family wanted that too.

A feisty woman with big blue eyes and red hair, Marcella had a regal presence. She played the queenly role, putting her arm out for someone to button her sleeves in the morning. In her mind she resided at the country club, and she expected full membership privileges. Her sparkly, mischievous personality had her tapping men on the behind on Rakhma field trips, then laughing madly. She could be an absolute lady or an outrageous flirt. She had strong opinions, and from the beginning showed signs of being aggressive and territorial.

A vacancy at Rakhma afforded Marcella the luxury of a being the sole occupant of a double room for a few weeks. When the second bed was filled, she became extremely aggressive. She was convinced the room was her private quarters and would push her new roommate out, yelling and shoving like a two-year-old. She extended her ownership to the bathroom. "Get out!" she would command, leaving frustrated toileters in her wake. Two minutes later she would forget the fracas she had created.

Her neurologist, Dr. Knopman, felt that her behavior would get worse, but suggested that the process could be slowed down with a small, very controlled dosage of medication. A little Haldol twice a day helped, but the bedroom remained an issue.

Marcella reached a point where she was so aggressive to her roommate that she could no longer be in a double room. The situation had to be handled quickly. It is one thing to train staff to dodge aggressive residents, but you do not want to put other residents at risk due to inappropriate behavior. There was a single room open, but not in the Peace Home. Marcella's granddaughter felt strongly that Marcella belonged at Rakhma, and said to do whatever it took to keep her at any one of the homes.

The manager of the Grace Home was apprised of Marcella's behavior and accepted her on a trial basis. It seemed iffy whether she would work out, given her aggressiveness. Manager consulted with manager to help ease the transition for Marcella, the new staff, and the residents of Grace Home.

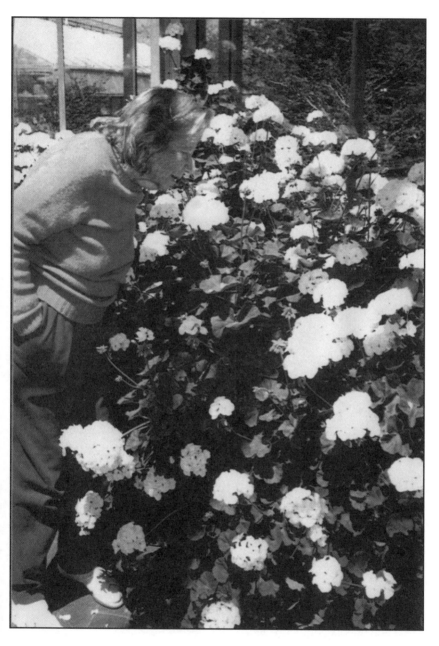

Marcella

"She has a way of hurting people's feelings, of lashing out verbally and physically, but she also has a sense of humor, reads the paper, feeds herself, and is not incontinent," said Winnie, manager of Rakhma Peace Home. "There are significant pluses that hopefully can be worked with in the new setting with a private room."

Marcella loved her private bedroom. After a period of adjustment, she seemed to be doing fine. Her independence fit into the household well, the private room alleviated the need to drive people out, the bathrooms were set up for use by more than one person at a time, and the suburban grounds were quite to her liking. She gave her family and friends tours of her new home (and bedroom) and could shower every day without cordoning off the whole bathroom.

Whose Reality?

When people become more confused as a result of their disease process, things that once came easily no longer do. For instance, an avid bingo player may begin to get agitated sitting at the dining-room bingo table. Because needs change from one day to the next, caregivers may need to intervene at times like this and usher the resident to a different setting.

Although the inability to express oneself usually comes on gradually, when you are used to finding the right word, understanding what other people say or do, and orienting yourself in your surroundings, these changes produce a great deal of anxiety. Just sitting by someone who is not able to express well, putting music on the tape deck, or giving a hand or forehead massage is very soothing and reassuring. Just holding a person's hand is giving them love energy. Our purpose is love. They feel it. Noises cease and things become much more peaceful.

Though changes can be hardest on family members, it is essential that family stay involved as their loved one changes. Letting go of the person they once knew can be excruciating, almost like death. Families don't want to say good-bye. They often want to buy time: "Maybe if you tried this or that Mom wouldn't lose touch so quickly." However, when a family member is involved, takes Mom out and spends time with her, they see that no one can control the changes that are going on. They begin to see that the things they are able to do with Mom now are not the same as the things they used to be able to do before.

Again, you have to pay attention, and this can be hard for families. Attention is what keeps us in the present. It's what gives us power in the moment to respond fully and appropriately. As people become less able and more disconnected, it's important to focus on whatever gives them pleasure rather than on our "reality."

For instance, Rakhma helpers spend time looking at cards and letters with Alice. She is now into a different reality and often wants to eat the card and chatter on about unrelated things. During the day she follows right behind the Rakhma helpers, almost connected at the hip. There are not a lot of activities one can do with her except to gently be with her. Helpers read to her from the Bible, especially the twenty-third psalm, and she clasps her hands peacefully as she listens. Those one-on-one activities are special times for both helpers and residents.

To embrace the reality of the person with Alzheimer's disease is especially difficult for family members. "That's not the way it was, Dad. It was a red car, not a black bicycle." Some families correct their loved one for a long time after their reality changes because it is hard to understand that Dad does not perceive things like everyone else anymore. However frustrating it is for the family to see this happen, it is equally frustrating for a person with memory loss to be corrected all the time. The corrections don't bring him back into our realty and, though well meaning, they tear down his self-esteem. Once the family sees that Dad is someplace else, they can come visit him in that place and listen and respond to him from where he is.

Different personalities respond to their memory loss differently, so of course they must be treated differently. If someone is in a high-anxiety place, you don't just send them in to join the others sitting in the living room. Instead, you or a helper spend a little time with that person. Some people have intense personalities that require a great deal of management. Others are more easygoing. They don't look for action or desire to stir it up. These people require less management but just as much attention and care to keep them stimulated and involved.

Working day to day with people who have Alzheimer's disease is extremely demanding. Many smaller settings are staffed around the clock with the same caregivers—what you might call a "ma and pa" model—and "ma and pa" burn out with the unrelenting responsibility that seven-day-a-week care is. Rakhma, though small, uses a shift-staff model that makes it possible for caregivers to work an eight-hour day, then go home and replenish. Thus, though some people do burn out, the shift-staff model enables staff members to approach each new day with fresh perspective and give residents the care and attention they need. Many of the staff love working in the shared-home model because, even though there is a lot going on, the emphasis is on quality time with the residents. There is time for fun, for one-on-one, something that's not available anywhere else. And new helpers come in with new eyes and new gifts, adding to the resources of those whose reality is changing.

When people are in a different reality, they might think there's a relative in the house. Or when someone goes out the gate, a resident may want to go too because she's sure she has to meet a friend for choir practice. Maybe a resident worries about the whereabouts of her daughter: "Have you seen Mary?" she'll ask over and over. In any case, these moments of waiting and watching often build anxiety. One thing that can alleviate the anxiety is to suggest looking for the person, though you wouldn't want to do this flippantly, over and over, as a ploy. It's simply a way to move the person from waiting anxiously to being in action and often they forget the original concern within three to five minutes, their attention being captivated by something else.

Again, it is the practice of ongoing awareness of what is needed by each resident each new day and responding to it that is the backbone of the Rakhma model. For example, even though Esther may be dressed warmly and the thermostat says 73 degrees, a helper, grasping Esther's cold hands, may bring her out to the kitchen for hot chocolate.

Esther is confused and has a hard time following what's going on around her, but one day I decided to ask her if she would like to watch a Shirley Temple movie. She just laughed at me, so I brought her into the fireplace room where the VCR was playing *The Little Princess*. She laughed at all the right times, but didn't watch much. It was almost like she was listening to a talking book. For someone who is usually pretty detached, she seemed to to be quite absorbed. She laughs easily and listens to what's going on. She can't walk, which frustrates her sometimes, but all in all she seems to be content.

With residents who are getting older and frailer, some days there is just no response. They won't eat much and look at you as if they mean to say, "This is it. I'm leaving." Helpers check the vital signs, and if they are below normal, call family. It may flat out look like their last day; then all of a sudden they look up and smile, ready to be with you again. And we are ready to respond to their living as well as to their dying in whatever way we can.

In addition to memory loss, Alzheimer's patients suffer many of the usual physical impairments associated with old age. They can't get around easily because they are stiff, can't see or hear well, need to use a walker, or any number of other things. Especially in the winter people are indoors more, and the primary questions become, "How do you provide stimulation? How can residents experience the expansiveness of life within the house?" Often simply changing where a person sits gives them a different view of their surroundings. Holding rocks from Lake Superior's North Shore, or seashells from the ocean, or tree bark or moss from a nearby woods brings the larger world of nature indoors and connects residents directly with the spirit within that longs to touch the earth.

One day when Lynn was over at Rakhma doing her mother's hair in the second floor kitchen, she remembered that the ladies had been having orange juice downstairs.

"I'll go downstairs and get the juice, Mom," Lynn offered.

Hard of hearing and quite advanced in her memory loss, Dorothy replied, quite sure of herself, "There are no Jews downstairs that I'm aware of."

Later, sitting under the hair dryer, sipping the juice that Lynn had retrieved, she was traveling the ocean on a ship to Norway and worried if she had registered for a room.

It is hard to see your loved one anxious, disoriented, upset, lost in their own world, and inhibited by physical impairments. But it is their world, sometimes replete with humor and often transformed by the simple act of acceptance.

How to Decide Where a Person Should Be

Although Rakhma is not a medical model, when people become weaker staff members keep a twenty-four-hour watchful eye for stroke symptoms or other health problems. Good follow-up is possible through careful documentation of changes in the log books and CNA's reporting to house managers and to the supervising nurse. However, some families want precise charting as you would find in a nursing home. It is really a matter of training families about the difference between shared-home care and nursing-home care. There is less structure in a shared home, fewer rules and less stringent procedures. There is more give and take, as in one's own home. That is what appeals to people. To get nursing home charting one must go to a nursing home. It is a different animal entirely.

Marlene was a wonderful woman with a twinkle in her eye who loved parties. If there was one, she was the life of it. She was driven to be on her feet all the time, simply couldn't stay still, and started to fall more and more often. She would trip over people's feet or the legs of chairs at Rakhma

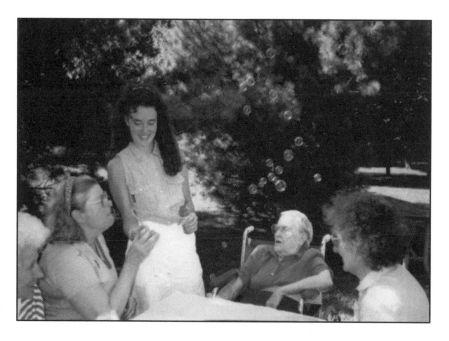

Blowing bubbles with Michelle; Esther in wheelchair

Grace. If there was someone in her way she would push them aside and keep going, causing hard feelings and fights. After trying a number of things including medication therapy to help her slow down, nothing worked except being with her at all times, sitting with her, asking her to wait, and helping her walk when she needed to go somewhere in the house.

One day I said, "Just sit with me for a while," and motioned her over to the couch. She sat, but a big tear came out of her eye. I saw how hard it must be to sit when your body wants to move. I also saw what it was like for our helpers to deal with those needs.

Besides, with other vulnerable adults in the home, her difficulty with balance was a big issue. Someone else could topple over with her. After trying everything, we recommended she move to a nursing home. We didn't want her to go, but it just wasn't safe for her to be here. We didn't want her to break a hip or hurt someone else inadvertently.

Safety is a primary concern when deciding whether it is appropriate for a resident to stay. These are the things we look at:

- The resident's safety: Are they falling? Do they need more than one person to transfer them as they need more care? Is the structure of the house right for them if they can't get down or up stairs? Is their behavior such that they can't be in a regular home setting; i.e., do they do things like eat lipstick, soap, or things that are not locked away?
- Other residents: How does the resident's behavior affect others? Is it upsetting? Do others have to defend themselves? Are the other residents becoming frightened of this person's temper outbursts? Are they at risk because of this person's behavior?
- Helpers: Does this resident require more care than staff can provide without depriving other residents of the kind of attention that is part of the Rakhma philosophy? Is the extra time and attention the care of this resident demands breaking down the morale of the staff? Is this resident's care becoming too stressful for the house manager?

Other reasons residents leave Rakhma are:

- Medical concerns that require skilled care under a medical model.
- Behavior that becomes unmanageable.
- The resident needs a first-floor bedroom and there is not one available.
- Funding. Residents usually come in to Rakhma home paying for their own care for some time. When people run out of money, alternatives need to be considered.
- Dying.

In exploring whether to become a resident of Rakhma, some families find that their loved one is not a fit, or that he or she fits in the home for only a short time. Even though they may not fit at Rakhma, they are helped, through meetings with our nurse, to find where they belong. Even though a resident may only stay a short time, they relax at Rakhma and are loved in a way they may never have been loved before. Rakhma is a transformational place for some families, giving them alternatives and time to think. One of Rakhma's gifts is being open to changes and helping others to be as well. Changes aren't easy, and are often painful, but an open heart, which is what Rakhma brings, touches and helps heal.

Helping Families Cope

Some Rakhma residents arrive when they are at a relatively independent stage. Very subtle changes, such as losing track of keys, missing appointments, forgetting the time of day, or not remembering names of children, have been occurring gradually over time.

Sometimes families want help in assessing what the next move is. Will assisted living work? Mom could still be independent, they reason. The Rakhma nurse looks at these questions: Are they starting to wander? Are they leaving the stove on? Are they isolating? If those things are going on, then assisted living most likely won't last. The big thing is the isolation. Mom's still going to be in an apartment by herself. If she's scared, especially at night, she will go out in the hall and look for other people.

In the last couple of years assisted living has changed appreciably. It now recognizes that as people age and change, they need more help; otherwise they cannot maintain their little apartment. You can contract with assisted-living facilities for cleaning help, bathing help, and any other help you need so you can stay longer. Then, of course, the rates are right up there, compared to the cost of twenty-four hour shared-home care, but without the continuity of a familiar staff being present at all times. Certainly, though, there is a place for assisted living. Our nurse's job is to look with the family at what would be best for their particular situation. Any move will often drop a person with dementia down two levels of functioning, then they will usually come up a level again after they adjust.

Isolation is usual with Alzheimer's disease. Memory loss is embarrassing. The person no longer remembers how to play cards, so they refuse to play. They don't remember names, even of their good friends. They isolate to be appropriate. Most families apologize for their loved one not being more social. At Rakhma, residents are drawn together. Because of their memory loss and inability to sustain what we think of as normal relationships, they don't usually socialize, but they do mingle. There are others worse off than they. At home, in their old surroundings, because they don't function normally anymore, they are the one who needs help.

Often in a home like Rakhma, it is a comfort to see others who are more frail. "I'm not like one of them," the resident feels. Staff says, "Could you help us?" They feel useful again. At home they need help. At Rakhma, even frailer residents feel they can provide help.

Some families have been to the Alzheimer's Association and know a lot about memory loss. Others, for any number of reasons, be it fear of facing their own aging, fear of loss, frustration, or denial, have not addressed the real causes of their loved one's changes and how to best cope. Dr. Knopman says there are diseases that are much more painful for the patient, but probably none more painful for the family than Alzheimer's.

According to Nurse Shari, "The biggest change every family has to go through is going from our reality to theirs. It is a grief process. 'This is a disease. Mom's not going to get any better. I have to change.'

"Some family members are frightened that they will have their power taken away. They don't want to think about what could happen to them if they had memory loss and became frailer. They want the person back as how the person was. But the truth is they don't have their old mom, and the question is, 'What can we do to make this mom more comfortable?'"

Care conferences provide families an opportunity to talk with the house manager and the nurse about what is happening, both to the resident and with family members. The conferences include not only the practical issues relating to the resident's needs, but concern for the caregivers as well. When asked how she was doing, Ollie's wife burst into tears. "No one ever asked me that," she sniffled. "They ask how Ollie is, but not about me. It's been so hard." Giving so much time and attention to the patient, the caregiver's personal life and needs get lost. It is a relief when someone understands the burnout, can lend support, and is willing to work together on the next step.

At first when a resident comes in, families don't know what to do. Should they hover about, call, take Dad out, not come for two weeks? Because each resident has different needs, there is no blanket statement. As families work together with the nurse and the house manager, trust builds, and trust is the basis for creating a solid care plan that includes the needs of the resident and the needs of the family. In one case there were six children, four in the area who were more involved with the prospective resident and two out of state who were creating problems by trying to direct things by phone. This tore the family apart. Nurse Shari's primary question was, "What can we do to cooperate?"

At one time Shari might have attempted to mediate over the phone. Then she learned that it's a matter of getting everyone together, finding out who's in charge in the family system, who has power of attorney. As mentioned before, if the family dynamic is understood, even if it is unconventional or dysfunctional, cooperation can often be achieved.

In one resident's case a brother from another state came out of the woodwork insisting he would take care of his sister, who was being moved to Rakhma. Shari encouraged other family members to let him try it and see how it worked. He soon discovered how far into her memory loss his sister was and what a huge task he had taken on. Once he saw the magnitude of the problem, and that he did not have the resources to cope, he was able to look at practical care options with the other family members and come to some agreement. It is often those who deeply love the person with memory loss, who still see them as they used to be and haven't absorbed the impact of the gradually worsening changes, who find it hardest to consider the need for full-time care.

Once families agree on a care plan, they are encouraged to think positively. Be aware of what the loved one enjoys. Do they relish maple nut ice cream? Bring some over or take them out for a sundae. Do they love a movie? A cup of coffee? A walk outdoors? A ride in the car? A foot massage? They may or may not still enjoy the things they used to. They may find pleasure in new, simpler things. Be aware and focus on those things. Those are the special parts of the person that you can relate to in the present.

There are families, too, or family members, who can't accept change, back off, and stop seeing their loved one altogether. This is not usually the case, but it does happen. It is not only a loss for the resident, but staff, as willing as they are to fill in and provide a family-like atmosphere, cannot take the place of daughters and sons, family and friends. It is a loss for the household as well.

What to do when a loved one becomes very ill is addressed right away when a family member comes to Rakhma. Some residents have living wills explicitly stating their wishes regarding extraordinary measures should they face a life-threatening situation. In other cases the family has to make those decisions. Some people want full code—do everything possible to keep Mom alive. One woman said, "Nurse, I want to live forever." Pay attention to the person who is ill and the wishes they express, even if they don't have a living will.

Living wills are a very useful tool. Doctors are trained to preserve life at all costs. Many of them still find it foreign to allow a person their leaving. When the doctor says, "You mean you don't want us to do more?" the family who has decided not to resuscitate or take extraordinary measures often feels guilty. If there are already orders or a living will, the Rakhma nurse can remind them that they are following the will and keep them from second guessing themselves.

In the beginning, we pussyfooted around the DNR/DNI (Do Not Resuscitate/Do Not Intubate) issue because it was so hard for families to put the person in a home in the first place. Shari and I found that it's important to talk with families up front. They take a tour of the home. We see their mom or dad or get an assessment from a qualified person in the city or state where they are now. As they fill out consent forms to go on outings and other admission forms, we include the DNR/DNI forms. For some people, it makes sense. For others, it doesn't. If they are not interested, we write that in the records.

If the family has not filled out DNR/DNI forms, we bring it up at other care conferences. When it looks like Mom or Dad could be dying, we talk again with the family. Most families, as the resident's health declines, do want DNR/DNI.

Care conferences are held at the request of family members, when there are conflicts within the family, or when family members' expectations differ from Rakhma's care.

So many times a family member has an expectation for a loved one, such as where she should sleep, instead of seeing what the person really needs. Clara sleeps in a recliner in the living room now because she has become disoriented and fearful in her bedroom. Her family understands the change and is okay with it. Other families can't see their mom or dad sleeping on the couch or somewhere other than in their bed, even though the person feels more secure there and can get their needs met.

"Mother has to have a private room," say some families. But Jean, for instance, had grown to love her shared downstairs room. Even when a private room became available on the second floor, and the first-floor space could have been filled easily with a less ambulatory resident, Jean's needs came first. It was not just a matter of ambulation or family preference, but of psychological well-being. The issue for Jean was not so much whether she was in a private room, but how she felt about where she was. The family understood and agreed to let Jean stay in her little shared nest.

In some cases the changes a resident goes through are unexpectedly beneficial. As her memory failed, Lynn's mother, Dorothy, always fiercely independent and strongly opinionated, began to allow hugs, foot massages, hand holding, and time for walks. In the past she had definite ideas of what she expected of her children, and she had a hard time letting them do things for her, but in her disease she became more vulnerable, softer, and though more anxious and repetitive, she allowed her children to be with her in a way that they were not able to be when she was "in charge." For Lynn, anyway, along with the sadness of saying good-bye to the old Dorothy, there was a sweetness in being allowed to love her mom in a new way.

Change is not an easy game. Changes are continuous, but not worth getting bent out of shape about. I had no idea this is what this work would be like. I had no idea it would entail so much paperwork and so many changes. Here I am over sixty years old, and I thought once we got something in place, it would stay that way. But it never does.

If there are changes in our residents, we always notify the family members. If the doctor calls us about a finding, we call the family immediately. If a new person is a smoker, since Rakhma homes are smoke free, we talk with the family about that.

Residents have creative ways of getting cigarettes—out of helper's purses, from a grandson, etc. Quitting smoking is a big change, not an easy situation, but with memory loss, a resident may burn holes in her clothes or set something on fire. These and other changes demand that staff call the family right away to let them help find an acceptable way to take care of the situation.

All the house managers walk a fine line when it comes to informing family members of changes or issues. They don't want to panic anyone, but they are committed to keeping them informed about behavior, health, and well-being. They approach change as an opportunity for new growth, even though at the time, addressing it may not be easy.

To Keep in Mind...

- Alzheimer's disease is a disease of unpredictable changes.

- Gentleness in handling change is required when working with people with Alzheimer's disease and dementia.

- To work effectively with Alzheimer's disease, the caregiver must pay close attention to what is going on in the present and dance with it. What is required at this moment may be different from what was required yesterday or an hour ago.

- It is life enhancing to respond to the reality of the person with memory loss, not try to get them to see our own. I have to change my position to be there with them.

- Family involvement is important even if changes in the family member who has Alzheimer's disease are stressful to deal with.

- Shift staffing helps keep caregivers fresh so they can better respond to the changing demands that are a part of caring for people with Alzheimer's disease.

- Sometimes diverting the attention of the person with memory loss helps alleviate their anxiety.

- Safety is a primary concern when deciding whether placement or a continued residency in a shared home is appropriate.

- Changes in the resident are always communicated to family members.

- Care conferences called by the family or the shared home staff help families and staff stay in communication, stay abreast of changes, and make appropriate decisions.

CHAPTER 6

Are We Having Fun Yet?
Activity Charts and Daily Living

It's hotter than Dutch love!
—Betty's favorite expression when she was having a good time.

Friends no longer move away. They die. A life once filled with work, bridge, golf, crafts, and studies is punctuated now only with daily "Jeopardy," meals on wheels, and a phone call from a son or daughter. The old homestead is no longer a support; it is a demand that can't be met.

Watching Mom or Dad live in an increasingly small world void of stimulation often prompts families to consider a shared-home living arrangement that would provide new friends and meaningful activities. Even if the move into a shared home is triggered by something else such as a fall or the inability to care for oneself, family members want to know, "Do you have an activity chart? In a time of change and loss can you bring some fun back into our loved one's life?"

Rakhma tried having activity charts. After all, it is a home that provides care and most care models use charts. It is an accepted practice, one that lends credibility to the overall care plan. You can see it right up there on the wall. But as in all areas of the care Rakhma provides, staff keep coming back to the philosophy of love, and you just can't chart that.

The unique feature of many activities at Rakhma is that they are part of the life residents left behind, occurring in the flow of the day, taking into account individual needs. It is a real joy to see people becoming host or

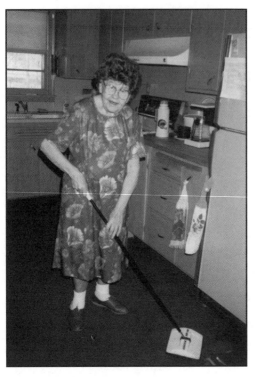

Clara doing her morning chores

hostess for the house, to greet visitors and offer them a cup of coffee. Or maybe someone enjoys grocery shopping, working in the yard, or running an errand with a staff member. All the houses have people who love to be involved in the kitchen, wiping down the counters or clearing the dishes. It's important that they feel at home and that they are free to do things they enjoy, are familiar with, and are still able to do.

Rakhma has found that anything residents do or are involved with is their activity at the moment. Shifting the focus from doing an activity "for" the resident to one of doing an activity "with" the resident or allowing them independent involvement stimulates wellness. Staff and family members are challenged to be creative, flexible, and willing to engage residents in activities of all kinds.

Ernest Meili was born in the French-speaking part of Switzerland in 1895. After his parents died when he was very young, he and his brother were raised in an orphanage in Zurich. He came to America in his early twenties, at first working as a farm hand in Kansas. Later, he enrolled at Wesley Theological Seminary, but he had some disappointing experiences which turned him away from Christianity.

He came north to Minneapolis where he attended the University of Minnesota and became a county probation officer. Eventually he was appointed Chief Federal Probation officer in Minnesota and remained in that position for several years. At Rakhma, he occasionally felt it was his job to check residents' pockets and purses for contraband.

His main love was for his family—wife Olive, daughter Jeanne and son Jack—followed by his love of gardening and fishing. Often, at Rakhma, he would go outside in the fenced backyard to rake or pull weeds. His daughter, Jeanne, who shared her father's love of gardening, came by frequently to plant and tend flowers with him. Ernest always enjoyed a good cigar, and every afternoon when the weather was nice he took his Havana out on the deck, surveyed the garden, and savored a good smoke.

Hilda had always loved to cook for her large family; she still tossed a mean salad in the Rakhma kitchen. She would hum merrily as she chopped her veggies. When Hilda's salads were served at dinner, it gave her great pleasure that staff and some of the residents could always recognize her special touches.

When she wasn't in the kitchen, Hilda liked to crochet colorful afghans. She kept her bag of yarn and her work in progress by her chair in the sunroom to show visitors.

Zeke, Alice's gray poodle, considered himself her guard dog, snarling at startled visitors and staking out her bedroom against intruders. When Alice died in 1990, staff weren't sure what do do with feisty, snarly little Zeke, but after a week of despondency, Zeke mellowed considerably and adopted the whole house. He became everybody's pampered pet. As he aged he had a medical sheet just like everyone else; he got his pills at designated intervals and he had special soft food because his teeth were bad. Until he died, there was even a cost of living for him under "Miscellaneous" in the Rakhma annual budget.

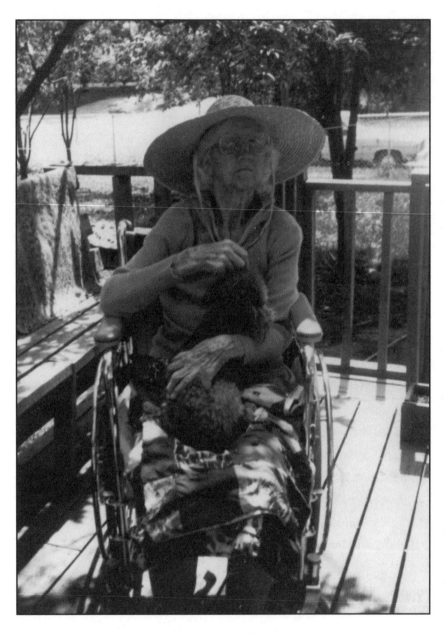

Alice and Zeke

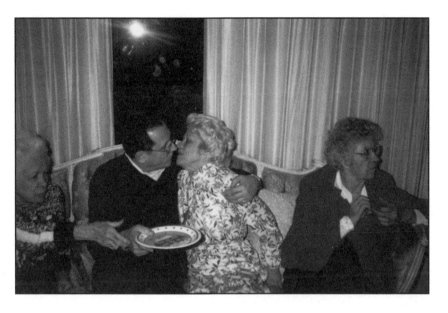

Helen, Kevin (Betty's nephew), Betty, and Hilda

People can have a good time if they can just laugh about something. Fun is a natural outcome of the touching, affirming, and appreciating that is part of the Rakhma model. The fun is in the spontaneity of playing a game, telling a joke, or singing a song. If one person starts laughing, the others will laugh too. It's infectious. Pretty soon everyone forgets the joke, but the laughter goes on and on.

Some residents with dementia have a need to take their clothes off. We try to take it in our stride and, at the same time, make sure we get the person to their room where they can be in the buff without embarrassment before getting dressed again. The sight of someone undressed in our midst is startling to those of us who live in the "real" world, but we realize that to someone with dementia, nudity now may feel perfectly natural.

Betty became known as "The Bra Artist." She could get out of her bra faster than a speeding bullet, a feat that always got fellow resident Paul's attention. No matter how many layers she had on, at least once a day Betty managed to pull her bra down the long sleeve of her turtleneck and out the cuff. One day, while on a drive, the house manager glanced over to the passenger side, aghast to see that Betty had not only removed her bra, but her shirt too.

"Betty, the cops will stop us!" she chided. "Here's a jacket. Please cover up."

Another time, during a staff meeting at the dining room table, Judy looked up to see Alice zipping by in her wheelchair stark naked except for Zeke, the poodle, on her lap. It seemed as though she just needed to ask someone a question, so a staff member excused herself from the meeting and graciously wheeled Alice back to her room, promising to spend some time with her after the meeting ended.

A lot can be said for paying attention to people as individuals. Rakhma being a very small setting, staff can tailor activities to suit the person. For instance, morning exercises in each of the three homes include range of motion and ball throwing. Lenora, a resident who recently came in, is extremely physical, more so than anyone else in the house. She loves to throw balls, but she throws them so hard she frightens the other residents. Now, when she does ball-throwing exercises, she uses a very soft ball.

Since pool was always one of Lenora's favorite activities, her daughter bought a pool table for the basement so her mother could still play. When she plays pool, a staff person plays one-on-one with her, making sure the pool balls stay on the table. The pool table and the one-on-one time gives Lenora a sense of security and the feeling that there is a special space in the house that is just hers.

Babies visit regularly. They come in with volunteers, staff, or with the resident's family members. Residents would rather watch a baby than eat their midday meal, asserts staff member Seini, whose daughter was the house baby until she started day care in her second year. Picilla came to work with her mother from the time she was born. There are eight residents at Peace

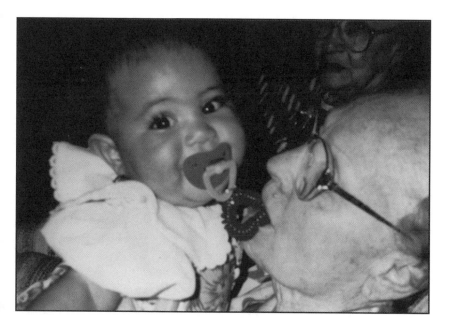

Baby Picilla Joy with resident

Home, so Picilla had eight house "grandmas" who participated daily with the little dark-eyed charmer as she grew from gurgling infant to fast-on-her-feet toddler. Cilla would pull herself up on Edna's walker, curious to see what was going on. Edna would laugh delightedly, sending Cilla off to the kitchen to see how lunch was coming.

"They just loved that baby," observed Seini. "Now that I think about it, it was an exuberant time for the residents. Everyone here had a pet name for her. Gertrude called her Prissy. Hilde called her Cookie and Tootsie. And Marcella called her Miss America."

Hilde once did child care for a living and liked to tell Cookie what to do. It felt familiar, gave her a sense of control, and made her feel useful.

The tenor of each house differs with the mix of residents.

For a while at Rakhma Home I, there were a number of lively dancers. Staff member Bob Kirkeide would tickle the old piano in the living room and residents would get up and dance. The present mix is a little more laid back, but they do love to sing.

The group dynamic can change quickly in the homes, either because residents leave and others with different personality types move in, or because of the progression of the dementia in members of the existing group. The Rakhma model provides the flexibility needed to respond immediately and lovingly to big and small changes so that activities enhance not only the resident's physical well-being, but their emotional and spiritual well-being as well.

In essence, the objectives of an activity at Rakhma are:

• To focus on abilities, not limitations

• A purposeful use of time and a sense of belonging

• An opportunity to support positive behaviors

• A tool to reduce or eliminate negative or unwanted behaviors

• A vehicle for verbal and non-verbal communication

As staff, volunteers, and family members learn and relearn, an activity should never be done for its end result alone. Activities are done for psychosocial, cognitive, and physical wellness. It doesn't matter if a resident sets the table the right way, or forgets what they are doing in the middle of serving snacks; what matters is that they are interacting with others and giving meaning to their lives. Almost all activities or tasks, even coloring with crayons, can be given dignity when the approach is supportive. Saying "Will you help me with this?" or "Let's do this for the Children's Hospital" often elicits participation.

In the Living Room
The Rakhma living rooms are spacious, inviting places with lace curtains and comfortable chairs. A lot happens there.

The Joy Home has a dancing group, inspired to shake a leg every Tuesday morning by a professional pianist who volunteers her time and talent. In the afternoon once a week at all the homes, dancers and wallflowers alike get refreshing foot soaks and don't even have to move from their favorite chair. A staff member soothes and massages feet with warm water and lotion, trims nails, and, again, has some nice personal time with each resident.

Morning exercises consisting of simple stretching for flexibility and ball tossing from person to person for eye-hand coordination take place in the living room. Often it is the place for impromptu as well as more formal meetings. At Joy Home the residents, most of whom were quite functional at the time, formed a residents' committee. In numbers there is strength, and they wanted more of a voice in the goings on of the household.

Many of the residents remember being active in clubs and organizations. At Rakhma Peace, as a new activity, staff decided to form a women's group; all women lived there at the time.

The meeting came to order. The minutes of the meeting follow:

WOMEN'S GROUP OF RAKHMA PEACE HOME MINUTES
January 12, 1993   1:30 p.m. at 4953 Aldrich Ave. So.

An election of officers was held. The results are as follows:
President . . . . Jean Fitzimons
Vice-President . . . . Hilde Conrade
Treasurer . . . . Gertrude Florence Mostrom
Secretary . . . . Dorothy Baskfield
Program Chairman . . . . Helen Mullen
Chaplain . . . . Edna Nelson

Absent: Evelyn Fewer (Day Care) and Isabel Friedman (napping)

Also present: Winifred Harris, Acting Home Manager, Elizabeth Manfredi, Acting Assistant Manager, and Leslie Kunzie, Acting Secretary

After the election of officers, a closing prayer was led by our chaplain, Edna Nelson.

Our next meeting will be on Wednesday, January 20, 1993.

It was decided that if Hilde interrupts the meeting any more that she will be fined 50 cents. If she asks Leslie one more time where her baby is, she will be fined $1. Hilde did protest this by saying she didn't have a paycheck but only lived on her Social Security check.

Jean was annoyed that people were telling her what to do, but graciously decided to be president.
Respectfully submitted,
Leslie Kunzie, Acting Secretary

The Dining Room Table

Some residents come in who are able to play table games like cards, bingo, or checkers. Siri, who is the house manager at Rakhma Grace, says, however, that "It's hard because everyone is at a different level. We've done bingo as a group, but you need more than one person to watch the cards, one person to call, and someone else to keep track of the whole group. We find that we are much more able to give a group of three or four the attention they need. Things get harder as the attention level of the residents isn't there anymore.

"Gladys is still fairly good at card games. 'Skippo' is her game. She needs reminding for counting once in a while, but she's still good at it. Alvin likes to play checkers, but he just doesn't get the gist of it. Then you just have to play along.

"One game we played that Esther and Helen used to love was the Little Fish game. Oh! They loved it! They'd try to catch the rotating fish and Esther got the biggest kick out of those fish pulling. They loved it! But they just can't do it anymore. As people become more advanced in their memory loss disease, they just don't understand it."

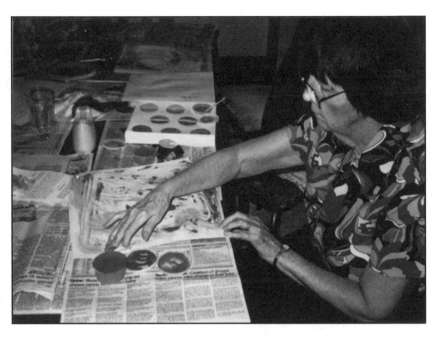

Pauline busy painting at the dining room table

The number one favorite thing to do is sit at the dining room table talking and laughing over a good cup of coffee. "Even the men like it," says Siri.

A copy of *The Clean Joke Book* supplements the easy conversation. The residents love the jokes and they read them over and over, laughing every time.

The morning paper is available for those who like to peruse it with a cup of coffee. *National Geographic* and *Reader's Digest* pique other residents' interest. Even though many of the residents can no longer read, they like to be read to.

The house gets *The Good Old Days* and *Reminisce,* two magazines that bring back memories with pictures and jokes and funny little stories about things like turning over outhouses and going to ice cream socials. Residents will try to remember related events from their own past as staff asks each one, "Do you remember going to an ice cream social? Was there a park where

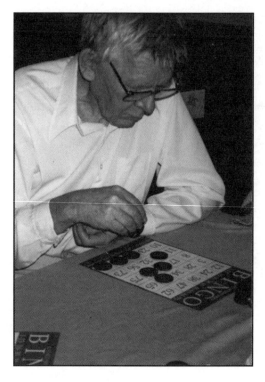

Alvin playing bingo

you grew up? Did you have an outhouse?" They love to remember and laugh. Dorothy did a little outhouse turning in her day—on New Years Eve—or was it Halloween?

This kind of reading and reminiscing works better at the dining-room table because people are sitting close together. The staff at Rakhma Grace have found that, even though the living room is comfortable, people are more spread out. The table acts as an informal focal point, drawing everyone's attention to one area.

There is a continuity provided that enhances resident's lives and triggers memories. To be able to remember stories of their own children, of being a child, or of growing up can be very stimulating for residents. Being able to speak what is in your heart is the heart of being alive. Staff members take time to listen carefully.

Outings

When I first started Rakhma, I was a wee bit idealistic. I wanted to include everybody all the time. Take grocery shopping, for instance. At first I would load three or four residents at a time into my old blue car to accompany me to the supermarket. It got to be amusing after a while. Our residents were taking things off shelves, leaving their carts, talking to strangers, and wandering

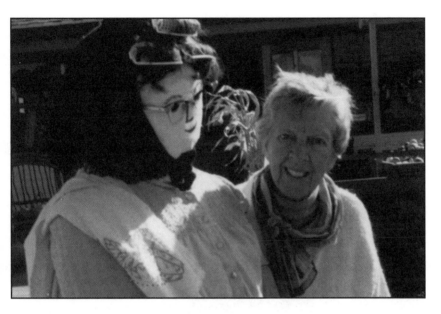

Scarecrow contest at Emma Krumbie's Restaurant with Helen

off thinking that the strangers belonged to them. I have discovered that taking one resident on an errand is quite enough.

Pam Boyce, the activity and volunteer coordinator, takes residents from all three houses on a special outing at least once a week in the Rakhma van. She tries to find places that are inexpensive so people can go out often. They might go to Perkins for lunch, or pack a picnic to enjoy at Fort Snelling State Park on the Mississippi River. She finds that just a simple drive to look at fall foliage or a stop at the Como Park Conservatory gardens is extremely satisfying to residents.

"I have found that the more simple the outing, the more enjoyable it is for all of us," she says. "The ones that are more successful are the ones that are purely for the soul: exploring the woods at Fort Snelling, watching the deer there, watching the birds feed at the Minnesota Arboretum, or just getting in the van and going for a ride around one of the many city lakes."

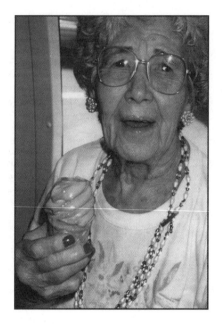

Edna with ice cream cone

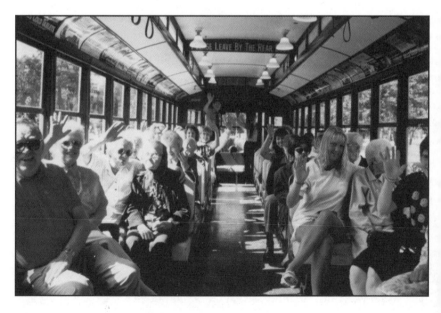

Lake Harriet trolley ride fun

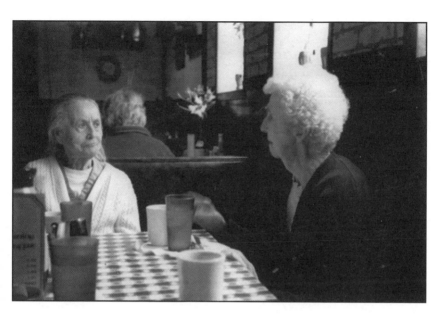

Luncheon out—Miriam and Emma

However, she, too, has refined how she conducts outings, having learned from experience that some things don't work.

"Sometimes taking residents on a bus for a special tour with a lot of people hasn't been as enjoyable when they are suffering from memory loss. They get anxious easily. It is harder for them to step up into a strange bus. We're always exploring, trying to find something that's fun and different for our outings that will work for people with their limitations."

That people with memory loss often suffer anxiety has to be taken into account when planning outings. We have to realize that, although we may think that going to the Scottish Fair at Macalester College would be fun, when a resident reaches a point where she doesn't want to get out of the car it could be that she feels more secure at home in her own yard. In the Rakhma homes you can walk out the door, breathe the fresh air, and sit among the flowers in the fenced backyard.

It could be that the resident is more content to be home in familiar surroundings. There is a point where some residents can no longer take part in many of the outings. When this happens, they are missed by the others.

Every month Pamalla sends a description of all the outings residents went on to family members. It might read like this:

> May 5—Gertrude, Kathryn, Dorothy, Hilde, and Evelyn enjoyed lunch at the Arboretum Tea Room.
> The cardinals especially fascinated Evelyn. Everyone enjoyed singing in the van on the way home.

Being that Rakhma is a small organization, Pam is able to send residents' family members photos of some events as well.

The Out-of-Doors

Each Rakhma Home has a fenced-in yard that residents can enjoy in the summer. Some like to play ball, just tossing it back and forth. There are yard games like horseshoes and ring toss, which appeal to some, but most prefer to sit quietly in the sun.

Helen at Rakhma Peace loves the outdoors. She is in and out several times a day. On cold or rainy days she looks out the window every few minutes. "Isn't it beautiful?" she exclaims, marveling at the angry sky or the newly mown summer grass in the yard below.

Seini says, however, that most of the residents at Peace Home are not the outdoorsy type. If you ask them "Do you want to go out?" they just say "Oh, mmm, uh." Because people need that fresh air and time outdoors to expand their world, staff have to take charge and say, "Come with me outside!"

On the other hand, Becky, the Joy House manager, relates this story:

"It was thirty-five degrees outside, the first warm day after several days of below zero weather. Kathryn wouldn't let herself be ignored. She needed to get out of the house! She appeared before me with her coat and boots

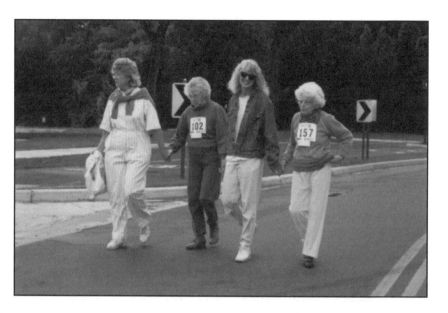

Senior stroll at Minnehaha Park
Shirley, Hilda, Krista, and Betty

on, so we went out for a walk. It was a sunny day. As we were walking, I picked up some snow to test how sticky it was. I threw a snowball at one of the big boulevard trees. They're so big even I can hit them!

"I gave Kathryn a handful of snow. 'Kathryn, see if you can hit that tree.' I threw and missed. Kathryn threw and missed.

"It had to be the oldest tree in Minnesota it was so big, but we both missed it. So as we walked along, we kept throwing snowballs at the trees and pretty soon we got pretty good.

"We had walked four or five blocks, watching and listening to the birds. It was just a beautiful day. We came down Wheeler Street in front our our Joy Home, and spied Kathy, our assistant manager, driving away. 'Kathryn, let's get her!' I said. We peppered the car with snowballs. Kathy laughed so hard she nearly went up over the curb.

"When we got back to Joy, we decided to build a snowman. We went inside. I bundled up the other residents and we all worked together to build two beautiful snowmen. It was fun decorating them with old eyeglasses, old hats, and scarves. There were leftover candy hearts from Valentine's Day, so we made candy-heart mouths."

What a memorable day it was!

Kathryn isn't the only one who loves walks. She can walk quite a distance, but others take just short walks down the block or even around the yard. A staff person always accompanies people on their walks, or a resident may accompany a staff member to the mailbox up the driveway. Then there is the Malt Shop down the street from the Peace Home—walking distance. This combines outdoor time with social time over giant hot fudge sundaes.

"I could never eat all this ice cream," Dorothy would protest. "Don't they have small ones?" Even though they don't have small ones, Dorothy would be the first one done every time, nicely fortified for the walk home.

Holidays and Celebrations

At Rakhma, residents are involved in helping with holiday preparations. They may help with Christmas decorating, make Easter tulips from crepe paper, or help bake a Thanksgiving pie. It is not uncommon to see a group of three or four residents pasting shiny paper rings together for a Christmas tree chain.

One day I joined a small group of men and women marching across the living room floor with their paper chain to hang it on the big spruce in the corner. The men in their nineties were having just as good a time as the women who, in the past, had traditionally done the decorating.

This kind of spontaneous participation helps alleviate the anxiety that many elderly people feel when they are not in their own homes. My intention is that people can be as involved in Rakhma Home as they were in their own home, even with their memory loss, for as long as they are able to do things. They are able to do a lot, even if it is just following each step of the preparations with their eyes. When staff are dusting, cleaning, fixing drapery rods, or painting, the residents love to watch all the action.

Every year there are special holiday outings like going to see the Festival of Christmas Trees in the auditorium of a local department store. It's a gorgeous, gala wonderland, colorful and artistically done. Gertrude particularly admired the glittering floral displays last year.

Dorothy's grandson volunteered to be Santa every year while his grandmother was still living. Short, redheaded Dan had his sleigh bells and sacks of red and green Hershey Kisses. As he sat down next to each resident for a little chat, he asked, "Would you like a kiss from Santa?" Santa's visit was a great excuse for a party. With coffee for the sipping, cookies resplendent with frosting for the munching, and carols tinkling on the piano, family members and residents mingled and laughed the snowy December afternoons away.

When a major holiday is not in the offing, the people at Rakhma make their own special holidays. On Resident Appreciation Day, family members and the whole household celebrate one resident's life. If the resident is of Italian heritage, the day will include mandolin music and steaming linguini. If they love to garden, flowers will be a prominent part of the day. Each resident has an appreciation day, and even if they are disconnected from their surroundings, the celebration goes on. Families come and share pictures and stories. Staff get to know the resident as a whole person, from his or her beginnings. The appreciation day fosters the respect that is the basis of the Rakhma philosophy.

Residents with dementia forget what happened at specific times, so it is fun to hear about them when they were younger, and to see their pictures and mementos. For instance, Ollie's Alzheimer's disease was at an advanced stage. He spoke very little, but his eyes told you a lot. His wife, Joy, came to his appreciation day with memorabilia from his past. Ollie had been an airplane pilot. Staff knew that, but to see photos and his pilot's cap reinforced

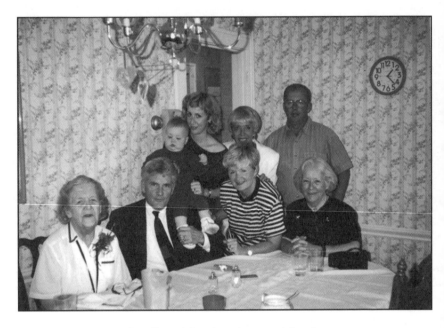

Family celebration, Jean and family

what everyone had only heard about, and it helped them relate more fully to the whole Ollie.

Everyone gets a cake and a corsage or a boutonniere to make Appreciation Day special.

Families are invited to use the Rakhma homes like they would their own, and use them for their own celebrations, as did Lynn's family when her mother, Dorothy, became too frail and confused to take her out to one of their houses.

Other celebrations at Rakhma include impromptu hat parties. Pam collects vintage hats, many of them in styles the residents wore in their heyday.

"We have these wonderful hats," says Pam, "and we laugh at each other wearing different ones. People pick out their own hats. We also have costume jewelry. We have a wonderful teacup collection, and we often, at the same time, have a tea party when we're wearing silly hats."

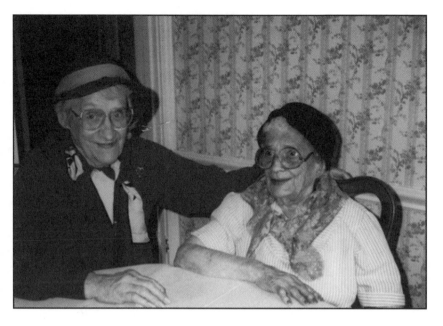

Gertrude and Hilde at hat party

Each home hosts a quarterly potluck dinner for volunteers, residents, and their families. People bring a dish, eat, mingle, and visit. Often there is special entertainment.

Body and Soul

Many of the most fulfilling activities are those that feed the soul. Even simple daily grooming rituals are deeply satisfying. On a Saturday or Sunday afternoon, staff might set up a nail-painting station in the dining room, with enamels from mauve to mango. Time together, touching, and attention engender a sense of well-being, as does feeling good about looking good.

Often after a shower, a resident will get curlers in her hair. The men might get a shave and a neck rub. At Rakhma Grace, a volunteer gives perms and haircuts. Sometimes a family member comes over to wash and set their mom's hair and spend a little time. Nothing feels better than a good shampoo and a touch of makeup. Some residents' families insist that their moms have makeup applied every day.

All the homes have prayer services, sometimes led by staff members and sometimes by an outside minister who will offer communion. Winifred at Peace Home leads prayers every week, complete with hymns. How functional the residents are impacts how much they can participate in services, but, according to Pam Boyce, they always welcome ways to express their gratitude to God. When residents hear, "Let's do a prayer service," most are ready to find a spot in the living room.

"Many add to the prayer reverent sentiments of their own. Some don't relate as much to the prayers as to hymns they remember. The words flood back and the voices rise strong from within," says Pam.

She observes that prayer and music are interconnected. When people with memory loss respond to the music, the sound and the beat trigger memories. Music was always in church, but it's more ancient than that. It's simple, she says. Music is the drumbeat of the soul.

Volunteers come in and play instruments for Rakhma residents. Some staff are musical as well, and share their talents, as do musically inclined residents like Paul with his mandolin. Even the people who can't speak are able to hum. They love the music.

Rakhma has a music therapist who comes in once a month, thanks to a contribution from the Honeybelles, a group of retired women from Minneapolis based Honeywell, Inc., who sing at Rakhma for special events. Rakhma has also received a grant for a storytelling project that connected the elderly with the community through the interactive medium of story.

Dancers come in to perform at the houses. The sound of clogging on the hardwood floors is riveting indeed, as is the synchronized movement and the colorful costumes. In each house, even as the mix of residents changes, certain individuals like to dance. When Miriam at Grace Home does her solo dances, I see it as an expression of her soul. When Norma

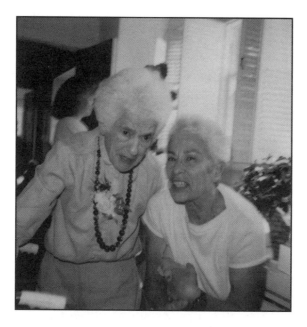

Appreciation day for Isabelle with daughter Sally

first came, she was quite mobile. She danced around the house like Isadora Duncan, waving her chiffon scarf.

"Where did this come from?" wondered her husband, Dick, who always thought Norma had two left feet.

However, the soul expresses itself, and some of us wait to dance until we cannot express in other ways.

Before Norma died, she couldn't verbalize at all. It was hard to see her essence, but knowing what her life had been like, we sensed that her spirituality was still intact. I can't believe anything different.

For the Mind

Elizabeth Manfredi is a fine artist who works as a caregiver at Rakhma during the winter and teaches classes and paints in France during the summer months. Sometimes she presents art-appreciation slide shows as part of her caregiving. She feels that several residents are interested in intellectual stimulation, particularly when placed in the context of spiritual and aesthetic growth.

One Saturday night she announced a slide show at 8:00 P.M. Once the women pried themselves away from the TV set, all four of the alert residents sat on the couch together to watch.

"They usually hate sitting on the couch together!" said Elizabeth. They were a captivated audience, and very gracious.

Recounts Elizabeth, "I felt that these women had open ears. The presentation was on landscape painting in the Middle Ages. I showed examples of the enclosed garden, and talked about its symbolism.

"The enclosed garden is a pathway for secular love, profane love, and also for sacred love. I showed pictures of the saints in the garden and the virgin in the garden. I tried to get them to think about how they live in an enclosed garden, and that even though it is enclosed, they can still feel a sense of internal growth. They can sit inside the garden and partake in that search for growth.

"I went into all this because I really think that, despite the Alzheimer's, there's a certain level in which their spiritual awareness is active, independent of their disease. There are also moments of lucidity that pop in and out."

Elizabeth feels that, although people with Alzheimer's disease have their special problems, as in any kind of teaching one's ability to stay aware and be aesthetically tuned is a discipline. It's essential to try to keep stimulating people—the "use it or lose it" theory. When people have lost their own drive or impetus toward stimulation, it's necessary to give of your own aesthetic discipline, moment to moment. This is what the residents respond to. According to Elizabeth, "You bring a part of yourself, your own personal self-discipline in the arts, or whatever activity, and watch that you don't get worn down."

It's a high demand job, to bring so much to the moment, and it's important to pace yourself, to come at it intermittently.

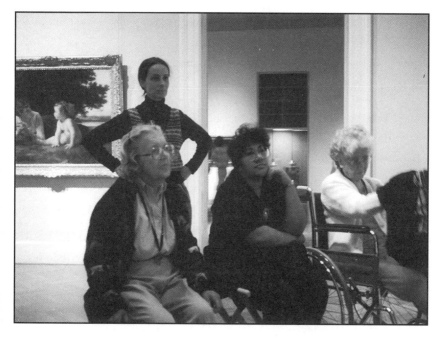

Elizabeth Manfredi (in back) at the Art
Institute with residents and Seini (center)

It all comes together again and again, making the original Rakhma vision of creativity, harmony, and love ignite newly every day. A recent summer afternoon in the Grace Home backyard had it all: cool breezes ever so slightly rustling the trees, residents sitting about the yard in lawn chairs, Edith and her son watering the early irises and feeding the squirrels, a volunteer chatting with Lenora. Enter Shirley.

Volunteer: "Lenora, tell Shirley what you just found."

Lenora: "What did I find?"

Volunteer: " A four leaf clover!"

Lenora: (Whistles with glee)

Volunteer: "See, it's over on the picnic table. I found one too."

Shirley: "Two four leaf clovers in one day. That's extraordinary!"

It's the extra in the ordinary that makes everyday life at Rakhma extraordinary. Are we having fun yet? You bet.

To Keep in Mind...

- You can't chart activities that occur in the normal unfoldment of a day, yet these are the activities that matter in the life of a person with Alzheimer's disease.

- Participating in the normal activities of a household, such as food preparation, laundry, grocery shopping, and grooming, gives residents a sense of belonging and spontaneity.

- For people with memory loss, stimulation is essential, but loud noise should be avoided.

- Always remember you are working with the essence of the person that is still intact.

- Laughter pleases the soul and brightens the day.

- Activities need to address not only physical well-being, but emotional and spiritual well-being as well.

- For those who are too frail to participate, observation is an important activity.

- Keep it simple. Do it with love.

CHAPTER 7

Small Really Works

I did not wish to live what was not life, living is so dear...
—Henry David Thoreau

When Rakhma Home opened in 1984, Alzheimer's disease experts agreed that you cannot care for people with Alzheimer's disease and the frail elderly in the same small setting. However, Rakhma did what the experts said would never work, and found that all but the most aggressively inclined residents blended well in this environment. Word spread that Rakhma was one of the few small settings that would take residents with memory loss; soon that became the focus. Here is what fourteen years of experience has confirmed.

A small home assures more one-to-one contact and stimulation. It is easier to keep track of residents with memory loss in a small home. A person can do "funny" things in a small home setting and still be an accepted part of the family. While in their own homes many Alzheimer's victims grow blank and out of touch, at Rakhma they gravitate to other residents, and, even in their forgetfulness, grow to care for them. Aggressiveness is handled with loving firmness and minimal behavior-altering drugs. Today there is agreement among more and more Alzheimer's disease experts about something that families and residents, the consumers of elder care, have known for a long time—that small really works.

Residents' family members agree with the consumer focus group findings discussed in Chapter 4, which call for basic conceptual changes when it comes to long-term care. These changes include less statutory regulation, more consumer choice, and risk management policies rather than risk elimination standards.

According to Colles Larkin, daughter of a deceased Rakhma resident, the whole approach to elder care needs to change. Her mother had spent some time in a large, well-appointed nursing home before she came to Rakhma, but, she says, "I was spurred to find something better when a staff member at the nursing home told me Mom was refusing to take baths and asked me if I would help. It was winter. I was wearing a cotton turtleneck with a wool sweater over it. A big tub stood in the middle of a room about twelve feet square with shelves on the wall, towels stacked, and dirty laundry bags in the corner. The aide got Mother totally undressed, rolled her into the tub, then filled it. Here's this poor frail little lady who could wear a cashmere dress in eighty-degree weather and be comfortable and there were no heat lamps or anything in that big room to keep her warm. No thought was put to this. I couldn't believe it.

"The dining room at the home had small tables and people were matched somewhat so they could socialize over dinner. But there were young people who worked there and evidently no one told them not to talk over the conversations of the residents. They would shout from table to table. It would have been very hard for anyone who is sensitive to sound. Dining there, to me, was a very sterile experience. You have to think about surroundings in a care setting.

"There was a bay window that looked over the inner court. There was not much to look at. Where the window was served as a corridor to the locked doors and beyond, and though there were places to sit, the chairs were high, hard-backed plastic lined up against the wall. It was the most efficient for cleaning, but not for people talking to each other in groups."

Colles had looked at options not only for her mom but for her husband's mother as well. She feels that "the whole program situation in nursing homes is not well thought out. There is not a lot designed for different levels of intellect and mental agility. There is a sensitivity level so often with big places that is not there.

"Places like Rakhma need to go forward," says Colles. "The small setting is better all the way around. I've been thinking about this and feeling guilt that I didn't find Rakhma sooner."

There are so few places like Rakhma that Colles' finding it at all was a tribute to her persistence and networking skills. She need not have felt guilty, but that is the natural tendency of family members trying do their best for a loved one while at the same time coping with the grief brought on by their failing health. Now Colles sees the bigger picture. She, like consumers across the country, feels our legislators need to be educated about solutions to the tangle of long-term care regulation, standardization, and paperwork so that home-care settings that don't exist could exist.

People-Centered Decision Making

One resident, Jane, has always helped other people. The oldest child in a large family, she took care of her many brothers and sisters. She raised children of her own and later in her life nursed and cared for her ailing husband until he died. As with many Alzheimer's sufferers, she is anxious a good bit of the time, but the home setting affords a familiarity where, even in her memory loss, she can look after other people and help with daily chores.

When Jane first came to live at Rakhma, she was given the sunny bedroom off the kitchen on the first floor because it happened to be vacant. When an upstairs room opened up, it seemed the natural thing to move Jane there because stairs were easy for her to navigate. The first-floor room would then be available for someone who was unable to climb stairs. However, volunteer coordinator Pam Boyce thought that might be a bad proposition, practical though it was.

"Even though she's only been here a short time, she loves that room off the kitchen and spends a lot of time there," observed Pam at a staff meeting. "The room is special to her. She's given so much to others all her life, I think she should have that room for her own."

From then on, the room was hers. In trying to work from our heart, we do try to think of each resident as an individual. What would really work for them? In a smaller setting, each staff member is more able to become intimately familiar with each resident whether they are direct caregivers or not. Pam made an astute observation about Jane and shared it with management in such a way that Jane's quality of life remained intact.

Many Ways to Include Family

We have many people we think wouldn't fare well in an institution. Viveca, a small Jewish peasant woman from Russia, was pushy and aggressive when she came in. "Tell me about your son," a helper would ask in an attempt to get to know her. "Why do you want to know?" she would spit back like a cobra poised to strike. Over time, staff saw that she needed her own space, yet she needed respect and community. She loved to dance, spinning to music and singing with a lilting voice. Viveca was given a loving welcome, time to adjust, and individualized, personal response to the needs that her forbidding behavior might have masked in any other setting.

She is still feisty, but she's mellowed a lot. We don't know what would have happened to her in a larger setting—maybe she'd be overmedicated, maybe get lost in the shuffle.

We had only one care conference with her family. Although we like to meet with family members regularly, if the family says they don't feel a need for a conference, we take it to mean they trust our care, and we accept that being in touch on the phone is enough. If we are able to get the resident to the doctor and if the family brings in clothes and other personal items, then we have to honor that. Not only do we need to work with the the resident's style and comfort zone, but we need to accept that of the family, too.

We had the meeting on a Sunday for the convenience of the family. The conference was about Viveca pushing other residents. We said she might have to move elsewhere if her aggressive behavior continued. The good thing about the meeting was that her family heard things about their mom they wouldn't have heard in a briefer, over-the-phone conference. Because the house manager was there, she could tell a story about how Viveca would put on her coat and insist on going out to feed the chickens. When she did this, one of the helpers would take her for walk, picking up on her need to go out and at the same time helping her to forget about the chickens. Her middle-aged son lit up. Having been just a young boy when his parents raised chickens, he was pleased Viveca could pull up that memory and engage with something she loved from so long ago. The family felt she was making some good connections with life at Rakhma and wanted her to stay.

We talked about ways we could work with her. She had a behavior medication. The dosage was changed and we were able to work with her behavior until she became more comfortable, or maybe her disease just advanced to where she became easier to be with. Though her fiery personality remains, no one would want her to go. Sometimes she bursts into tunes that another resident will pick up on. The two of them will sway and voice some ancient melody from deep within. Connections like this touch the core of the being and are invaluable.

We just had a family whose mother died in our home after being with us only a few months. We did hospice for her. We weren't sure our setting was the right one as she was tippy on her feet and we couldn't be with her every minute, but she cried all the time in the nursing home she had been in. The family wanted her to to have the kind of loving attention that they would give if they could be there all the time. She did have periods at Rakhma where she was weepy for a while whenever her family left. She relaxed, though, after she had been here for a few weeks. You could see her in the living room sitting on the couch with her head on another resident's shoulder. The family was happy to see their mom content.

The family was especially touched by their mother's life at Rakhma, and felt that her time here was a gift. As a memorial to their mother, they returned the gift after she died by donating money for a wheelchair ramp to be built at the Peace Home where their mother had lived.

A Funny Thing Happened

A person can do "funny" things in a small home setting and not cause a disturbance. Nurse Shari arrived at the Joy Home one summer morning as a helper prepared to take Alise for a stroll through the neighborhood. It was a day like any other, except that Alise had accessorized her left ear by placing a three ounce paper cup over it. Eagerly, she stood by the back door, smiling from ear to Dixie-cupped ear, waiting to go. Shari decided not to say anything, as Alise seemed so happy.

Right about the same time, the delivery man from the drugstore drove up with a prescription, which he gingerly handed to the helper, looking all the while at Alise out of the corner of his eye. A bit unusual, yes, but in a shared home there is room for residents to be just who they are. Shari didn't explain to the delivery man, but just gave Alise a big hug as she set out for her walk.

Alise is partial to paper products, says Shari. In the past she has greeted people with a toilet paper bow around her neck. Sometimes she pulls her hair back with toilet paper. What's not normal in the outside world becomes normal to the Alzheimer's patient. There has to be room for that. "None of us are normal," laughs Shari, referring to the Rakhma staff. "We know that. That's why we can work here."

Smitty had climbed to the top of the corporate ladder, but by the time he was in his late fifties, his memory got so bad he could no longer work. His wife took care of him until she couldn't handle him anymore, then moved him into a nursing home. It was a lovely place, but too confining for Smitty, who had kept fit all his life and lived to jog outdoors.

One day when Dick Wiessner came over to Rakhma, Smitty was in the family room with his wife, who was considering moving him there. Dick had known Smitty from being on church committees with him years ago. Though Smitty looked like a man in his prime, fit and lean, when Dick offered a handshake of recognition, he was full of talk but out of sync with what was going on. "Another young casualty," thought Dick, and his heart went out to Smitty's wife and family who were shouldering the tremendous responsibility of taking care of someone with Alzheimer's disease as he had done with his wife, Norma.

Smitty did move into Rakhma, where Dick saw him often when he was visiting Norma or helping out at the Grace Home. One of Smitty's daughters was delighted that someone from his past was around so much and asked Dick if he would take her dad out to lunch once in a while, somewhere where he could get a beer. Dick spent quite a bit of time with Smitty, getting to know him again in his memory loss, spinning yarns and talking men talk over beer and sandwiches.

"There was a young kid by the name of Sid who worked at Rakhma and who was great with residents," Dick related. "When I had projects I couldn't do alone, I'd ask him to help me. One day I decided to haul brush out of the yard to a dump about fifty miles away. 'Lets take Smitty!' I suggested. Sid agreed. At the dump he'd have some room to move. He'd be happy.

"We threw brush from the back of the van over the edge of a hole at the dump where they could burn it. One minute Smitty was standing right next to us, hemming and hawing. The next minute he decided to take off down the road. We thought he'd be okay just jogging a little while we quickly finished. But he was very fit and could go a long way in a hurry. We had to get in the van to catch up with him; then he wouldn't get in. Finally, we talked him into it. At home, not taking any chances on letting him get away, we drove right up to the garage door and parked so he would have to go straight into the garage when he stepped out of the van. He was too fast. He slipped past the garage door and started running down the road. He even stopped to turn and wave at us.

"We went after him in the van. Smitty ran into a cul-de-sac. We thought we had him cornered, but no, he ran right on by us, out down the road. We had a trailer behind the van that made it hard for us to make quick turns. He must have run an hour or so, but he kept on running. Sid and I decided to position ourselves someplace where we could keep track of him. We knew if he thought he was being chased he would run faster, and we didn't want to push him further physically than he was able to go himself. So we just followed him at a distance. He made a turn. We made a turn. Finally, Smitty went down a road and made a left turn. There was only one place he could come out so we went there and waited.

"We knew he was running out of gas by this time. He'd traveled quite a distance. I got out of the van and came up to him like I hadn't seen him for a long time.

"It was the Fourth of July. As Smitty approached, I saw that he had stopped along the way to pick things up off the road—cigarette butts, papers from firecrackers—he had a whole handful of things like that. I held out my hand. 'Smitty, how are you?' I said. 'Want a ride?' And that was it. He was glad to see me and climbed in the van."

Smitty loved to be outside; his family loved having him at Rakhma. After his adventure, they installed a sturdy, six-foot cyclone fence around the backyard that would make it possible for him to enjoy being outdoors as often as he wanted and still stay safely at home.

Usually in any Rakhma home you have one or two "bundlers," residents who tie things up in little bundles. It could be a bundle of breakfast toast, somebody's mail, napkins, or anything. Sometimes you might find things wrapped up in a towel. Everyone gets used to people doing this. If you ask the resident what it is, they may say they are getting a package ready to mail. Unless there's something you really need in that bundle, you let them have it to take around with them. The bundle has great meaning.

Residents carry interesting things in their purses, too. Along with pictures of children or grandchildren, jewelry, and makeup, they may have other people's mail, false teeth, or glasses. It's not intentional taking, but they like to squirrel things away. People with memory loss often don't differentiate between what belongs to them and what belongs to someone else.

Jean was forever carrying cups of tea to her room and pouring them out of her window. When winter came and the storm window was shut, she poured tea on the window sill. In spring, vestiges of frozen tea, cookie crumbs, and other miscellaneous treasures were found there.

Her daughter regularly discovered coffee cups under her mattress. Jean is definitely not the princess and the pea. Maybe she was trying to put together a tea set. She's such a hostess.

One resident had a habit of flushing her underpants down the toilet. She was such a lady that she would be embarrassed if she soiled her pants. While respecting the delicacy of the situation, staff put clean underpants on a high shelf in her closet. Now she asks for clean pants, and they can check the toilet or wastebasket for any she may have disposed of. Along with being attentive caregivers, staff have learned to be clever detectives and creative problem solvers as well.

Parallel dialogue is common among Alzheimer's sufferers. Some residents look as if they're listening, so absorbed are they in the conversation of the person sitting next to them. Their response may be lengthy, in the same friendly conversational tone as any parlor chat, but completely unrelated to what the first speaker was saying. This doesn't seem to bother either party. They listen, laugh a little, respond. "Is this your purse?" "Oh yes, Henry and I went there yesterday!"

One day two women, Myrtle and Sarah, who looked somewhat alike but were unrelated, were sitting on the davenport. Both carried purses, which they would routinely clean, pulling out their makeup, tissues, and family photos and putting it all back in again. One picked up the other's purse, went through all her pictures, and declared they were pictures of her

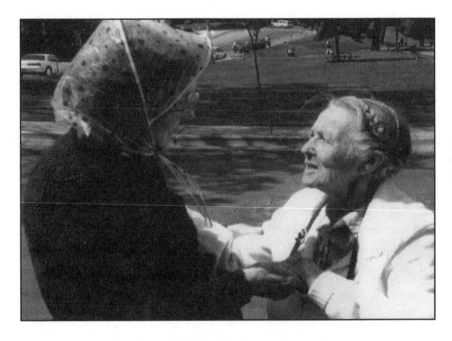

Connie and Miriam having a conversation

own family. The two of them were getting along beautifully and having a
wonderful time reminiscing.

"Remember how often we'd get together?" Myrtle sighed, pointing at
the people at the picnic table in the photo. "We'd do this all the time, Abby."

"Oh, ya," agreed Sarah. "But my name isn't Abby. My name is Sarah."

Myrtle didn't understand and called her Abby again. "I'm not Abby,"
Sarah insisted.

"Well if your name is Sarah, why did you let me call you Abby all these
years?" demanded Myrtle, miffed to be just now discovering this.

When a resident has a conversation which has to do with the reality
they are in, we reassure them. Someone might say, "Mother is coming," or
"A whole room full of relatives are coming. There's not enough food." We
reassure them there is a lot of food. All the relatives can come. There will

be enough. How do we know they're not recalling an event like that where there really wasn't enough?

It doesn't do any good to do reality orientation, especially if the resident thinks her husband is alive, or her mother or child. Just let them be, listen, comfort if necessary, or distract them. Take a walk, have coffee. Instead of telling them your reality, think, 'What can move them from their distressing thought?" Often, laughter is the ticket.

One day the chairlift to the second floor bedrooms at Rakhma Home 1 stopped working. Dick Wiessner came over to fix it. Almost as soon as he set his toolbox down by the lift, residents gathered around. Dick asked Betty where she lived. She gave the correct address of her home in Winetka, Illinois, where she thought she was.

"It was a typical day," commented Dick. Betty was charging around Illinois. Someone was fixing a resident's hair. People were in their different realities. Dick got the chairlift fixed and went to get the vacuum cleaner from the closet in the dining room to clean up. When he opened the closet door, boots and miscellaneous stuff tumbled out, overflowing their confines as if this were Fibber McGee's closet itself.

"By this time," reported Dick, "Paul is over on the couch grousing about the whole situation. 'What's he doing over there in the closet?' he's saying over and over, getting quite put out. I decided to have fun with it, even though I was thinking to myself, 'Isn't there a better way to arrange this mess?' I stepped into the closet and closed the door. I can hear Paul giving orders. 'Get that guy out of the closet. He's goofy.' I step out of the closet. Everyone laughs. Betty is holding hands with two gals. Linda, one of the helpers, comes out of the kitchen. 'What's going on,' she says. 'It sounds like a nut house in here!' 'We're going to a nut house,' squeals Betty, delighted. 'Let's go to the nut house,' everyone chimes in." Everyone was laughing and involved in the fun.

In a small home residents often sit three on the couch, physically connecting just because of the proximity the living room affords. Touching another human being is important, especially since people with Alzheimer's disease tend to isolate more if left to themselves. That's all we can do for people, sometimes: let them know we love them.

"You have such a smart daughter," a helper might say as he sits down next to a resident on the comfy sofa. "She's a wonderful lawyer. Your daughter's almost as good looking as you but not quite." That brings a smile.

One day Paul was upset to see Gerry, sitting across from him on a recliner with a throw over her lap, move around in her chair enough so that her skirt crept three or four inches above her knee. He yelled, "Pull her dress down," to whoever might be within earshot. A helper came over and pulled it down. Soon Gerry rustled around again. Her skirt again crept up over her knee. Paul yelled again for someone to fix it. "He was owly that day," said Dick, who was there involved in a project. "I tried to divert his attention, but he wasn't about to be dissuaded."

As Paul's outrage escalated, I came in. "Paul, are you out of sorts today?" I inquired.

"Pull her dress down," he sputtered.

"It won't matter that much, Paul. It's just a little knee showing."

Paul continued to grumble.

I plunked myself down on his lap, hugged him, and gave him a big kiss on the cheek that knocked his cap off.

Without missing a beat Paul looked up with a sheepish grin. "Put her there, baby!"

The first step is to sit together and be with the person. Telling someone with Alzheimer's disease to sit down and relax doesn't work. In addition to needing a sense of community, they need one-to-one time. It really doesn't take that much.

Flexible, Responsive, Individualized Care

In a smaller home, if you're running short on help, or if someone is late for a shift, you can manage for short time without being too stressed out.

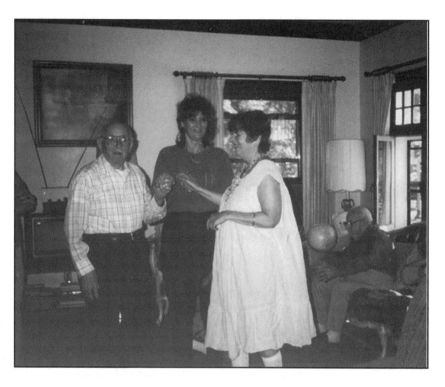

Paul, Linda, and Gerry dancing; Grampa
Meili playing ball in the background

In a smaller setting, even with one staff member missing for part of a shift, residents are pretty much guaranteed to have the attention they need.

The schedule can be flexible in a small home. If one resident, for whatever reason, needs more time, another resident can get up or go to bed a little later. One woman wants a bath every day and lashes out when she can't have what she wants. Staff gives her a certain bath time every day and gets her up earlier to use the tub.

With a nonmedical model, residents can be much more involved in household tasks. Whatever it is that they like doing, staff knows them well enough to call it forth in them and make them feel appreciated.

When residents are experiencing memory losses, staff in a smaller home can reinforce what the person can still do. This feels good to the resident. Some people forget how to do many of the things they used to enjoy, but they can do other, related things. For instance, at Rakhma, if someone forgets how to set the table, they may still be able to clear it. They are encouraged daily to do what they can.

In a small home there aren't many restricted areas. Two of the eight Rakhma Peace residents know where the business office is in the basement. They know they can come down anytime and talk to someone "in charge." At Joy Home, when Kathy, the assistant manager, is working at her desk, she invites residents who come by to sit down, sometimes giving them some "writing" to do. They enjoy being a part of the office hum. Almost all of our people would be in a secured area in a nursing home. They would have a lot less freedom of movement. Even going into another person's room and napping on their bed is accepted by the other residents.

Dr. Knopman didn't think our early resident May would work out in the home setting, but she did. She was most difficult, but we enjoyed having her around before she went to a nursing home because of aggressive behavior. She learned about being touched and hugged and kissed at Rakhma. She would still strike out, but afterward she would say, "I love you." Before she came to Rakhma, she never said, "I love you." She learned about love here.

You're not going to get many unflaggingly sweet, docile people. They wouldn't be in our homes if they didn't have special needs.

Rakhma plans activities that bring richness and variety to people's lives. When I go to a concert during the week, I am tired when I get home, but there is a richness in the activity that is different than coming home from work tired. That is why we have potlucks and some special, individualized activities during the week. At potlucks, sons and daughters become familiar with other residents and their families. "Hi, Betty. Hi, Jean. How are you?" Sometimes in the wake of special activities people are tired the next day, but they love it.

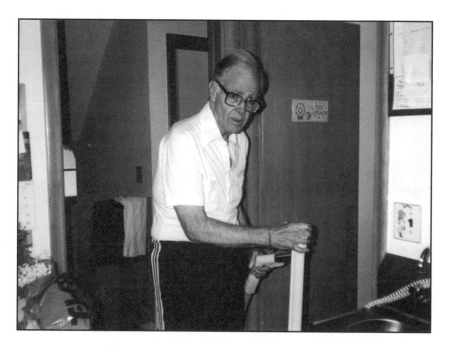

Waverly Smith helping with vacuuming

Barbara's breast cancer left her so depleted and depressed that she would sometimes fall asleep at the table. She had no desire to feed herself. She would sip out of a straw in a glass, but to lift the glass was too much effort. However, she was full of the dickens and could swear like a trooper. "You're such a great part of our family," staff would say. "You're a great person. Do you have anything you want to add?" "Thhhhht," Barbara would reply with a roll of her tongue. For a little special time, staff took her to see a five-year-old cockatiel named Beatrix that belonged to my granddaughter. The orange-cheeked bird with white feathers that went straight up was as full of the dickens as Barbara. "What a babe, what a babe," the bird would repeat as she danced in a circle, making Barbara laugh at its limping rhythms.

In many nursing homes there are a lot of activities, but sometimes staff members forget to encourage people, especially those who are frailer, to participate. You can have a lot of activities and still not have many people involved. It is important to plan things that bring residents together and that encourage laughter, even if it's balloon throwing, exercises, or walks.

However, everyone in the Alzheimer's community is in agreement that too much stimulation is hard on people with dementia. Noises seem louder. Din is upsetting. It is important that the person can be out where there is activity or retire to their room or go back and forth. Rakhma's goal is to minimize loud noises. In a smaller home there can be lots going on, but there isn't the noise of carts being pushed up and down halls or lots of people talking.

When there are tours, time spent in the residents' living areas is kept to a minimum. People who come through are introduced as friends, then are walked on through to meet elsewhere. We don't want to disrupt our residents' lives because of our needs.

A healthy daily menu is planned and served on a six-week rotation. However, each house manager responds to residents' individual needs. People with Alzheimer's disease frequently get thinner as time goes on. Added snacks, health drinks, and extra calories can somewhat offset loss of appetite and other changes in the body which exacerbate weight loss.

I love residents being involved in meal preparation, especially peeling vegetables. For some people, that is important work. Take a simple cottage-cheese salad. If they can't make it all, they may start by putting the lettuce down. Then a helper will prompt them to plop on the cottage cheese or do whatever keeps their attention. They love the recognition. They like to feel they are contributing something, that they are needed. "What would we do without you?" we say. "Can I give you a hug?" We tell them how special they are. I think I probably need those hugs more than they do.

A Home on Every Corner
Hilde raised her family and went to church in a neighborhood close to the Peace Home. Her daughter lived nearby and stopped in every day, often

with Hilde's great-granddaughter. Old friends and fellow church members came by regularly.

Hilde had been at Rakhma for four years before she died in her mid-nineties in 1996. Toward the end she needed total care, and got it with a lot of love from the helpers she knew so well. She dozed often, but still enjoyed sitting in a recliner in the living room during morning prayer services. Staff member Winnie always had a special, teasing relationship with Hilde, giving little punches in the arm back and forth. They continued to share that repartee, even as Hilde moved more and more into her own little world, looking up at the ceiling and talking to people who weren't there. I felt that she was having a lot of dreams that were real to her. Who knows if she wasn't having visits from loved ones who have passed on?

In a new paradigm of care, there would be a shared home for the elderly similar to Rakhma at the end of every block. Being in the neighborhood where they have lived much of their lives would give people a sense of home. The same stores, the same funny beauty shops, the same streets, the same trees—even in their dementia, people with memory loss sense the familiar.

When Norma moved into Joy Home in St. Paul, she was a half-block from the home where she and Dick raised their four sons. She would look out the window, rub her hands together, and exclaim, "Oh! oh!" She seemed to derive comfort from the scene outside. Until she became total care, she went to Arlene, the same beautician she had gone to for years. Though her memory loss got worse, she could still go to the same place.

There are duplexes for ten people and fourplexes for twenty people with memory loss being built at this time in Minnesota. The floor plans are good. However, I prefer individual homes in residential areas. I like homes that are already in the community. I like utilizing buildings that are already in existence. People have grown up in lots of kinds of homes—little, big, on a lake, in the city, in the country. Why not have more places reminiscent of one's own home, in the heart of one's own community?

To Keep in Mind...

- The small setting is conducive to observing each individual's behavior and needs.

- The small setting allows for flexibility in working with families.

- "Funny" behavior is included as a normal part of daily life. Residents can be who they are.

- The low ratio of staff to residents makes it possible to respond to challenging situations creatively without resorting to medication unless absolutely necessary.

- Due to proximity and seating arrangements in a small setting, there is a physical connection between residents that creates community.

- The nonmedical model that a shared home is allows for flexibility, less restriction of movement, encouragement to participate, and less overall clatter.

- Familiar, homelike surroundings comfort many who suffer from memory loss.

- A small home fits naturally into the community.

CHAPTER 8

We'll Be There 'Til You Die

The Continuum of Care

And did you get what
you wanted from this life, even so?
I did.
And what did you want?
To call myself beloved, to feel myself
beloved on this earth.
—Raymond Carver, "Late Fragment"
from *A New Path to the Waterfall*
(Atlantic Monthly Press, 1989)

Care does not have a beginning or an end, but remains always sensitive to the ongoing needs of the elderly and their family members. Like hospice, Rakhma aims to help people fully live their lives and their deaths.

The only reason anyone has to leave Rakhma is if they are harmful to other residents, are unmanageably destructive, become hospitalized, or can't afford to stay. If a resident leaves, staff people from Rakhma help him or her feel more secure in the move by bringing music and hugs to them in their new home, often up until their death. Being there through losses with residents and family members is an essential part of the Rakhma model. Staff, residents, and I often attend the funerals of residents who have died, and Rakhma hosts a memorial service as well for family members, staff and homebound residents.

Going to a Nursing Home: When a Resident Has to Leave

George, a seventy-year-old resident with bright blue eyes and a mischievous grin, loved to tease. When he tickled Clara's toes, she'd scream, "Don't,
don't!" but that just egged him on.

Up and about all the time, George would look closely at other residents
and try to read the expressions on their faces. One day he decided that Gerry,
who was by then completely nonverbal, and two others looked like they
wanted to get out of their chairs. Gerry sat in a wheelchair while the others
enjoyed recliners. George helped each one out of their chairs and laid them
very gently on the floor. Siri, the home manager, said it was obvious that, in
his mind, he was doing what he thought was needed: his fellow residents
wanted to go somewhere and he would help. Having just been in the living
room moments before and finding all to be well, she was astonished to walk
in again and find George in the process of laying the third person on the floor.
He was a quick one! His "helping" of the other residents like that happened
just once, but it was a red flag signaling staff to watch him very carefully.

George liked to put all kinds of things in his mouth. He would go into
people's bedrooms, take lipsticks and perfume bottles out of drawers, and
eat or drink the contents. He would drink liquid hand soap or chew solid
soap like a candy bar. Buttons and chips from board games went into his
mouth, too. Some people with memory loss do put inappropriate things
into their mouths, but being a little slower, they can be caught and redirected. George was fast. He'd get a grin on his face like a naughty boy saying, "Got one on you!" He was very cute, but he put himself at risk.

Once he slid a lawn chair up to the six-foot cyclone fence in the back
yard of Grace Home and climbed over. The helper who saw him leaped
into her car and met him standing by the road thumbing a ride. Though he
was grateful for the lift, he didn't recognize the helper when he climbed
into the car and gave her his family home address. When she brought him
back to Rakhma, Siri explained to him how dangerous his adventure had

been. "You could have been killed, George. Don't ever do that again." After that, George cautioned residents in the backyard, "Don't get on that road. It's dangerous." It's unusual for someone with as much memory loss as he had to take heed from even a dangerous situation, but he never went over the fence again. We really thought he'd try it again, but he knew Siri was in charge and she must have made quite an impact on him with her hand gestures and I-mean-it voice.

When George's compulsive behavior continued to accelerate, it became too stressful for staff members to monitor him all the time. George took so much supervision that other residents were getting less attention. Shari, the nurse, sat down with the family to talk about placing him in another setting. There comes a time when we just have to let go, to let the person move to another setting that's safe for them.

When George went to a senior care center, staff from Rakhma visited several times. Even though he could barely remember his own family anymore, we could laugh and talk and kid him and tell him what a beautiful grin he had. Over coffee and cookies we would talk about things from the past.

Visits like this are made on work time by house managers and assistant managers to most residents who leave Rakhma for another setting. It is part of the Rakhma commitment to continuity of care. I find that helpers frequently visit on their own time, too.

Rakhma keeps people like George longer than some smaller settings do. We want to determine if the compulsive behavior is a stage they'll pass through. We pay close attention with staff as we monitor a resident like him.

Very often families want to keep their loved one with us, even with the risks involved. But if a resident does get hurt, the family feels guilty. We keep asking the family to look at how they might feel if something happened, to keep them aware of the real situation. We respect families' desires, but if a resident's situation becomes dangerous, if a person is very tippy, misses steps, or we have to keep a helper with them at all times to watch them, we recommend they go to a setting that is better equipped to work with their needs.

After George made the transition into a nursing facility, Rakhma's visits lessened as the new staff took over. Even after residents have left and have acclimated to a new setting, the Rakhma staff and I like to have family members call and tell us how former residents are doing. When they have to leave us for whatever reason, we try to do that follow up. We are always interested in hearing about our "family." It would be our joy to hear about former residents' lives regularly.

Olga's Transition

At Rakhma, always the first response is to accommodate the resident's personality and needs and to work with their dementia.

Many people with Alzheimer's disease will go to the bathroom at night in their wastebasket, and even move it into the closet. When this happens, staff will move a commode into the person's room and usually this works. Olga quit using her wastebasket after getting a commode in her room, but she couldn't just leave it at that. Always creative, she enjoyed shaping her bowel movements into little balls, wrapping them up, and tucking them into the cups of her clean bras in the dresser drawer. Once she arranged some in a small box, like chocolates, and wrapped them like a gift. What a surprise someone would have gotten had staff not peeked into the box!

Olga could be very sweet with her Scandinavian accent and big smile, but as her Alzheimer's progressed she could suddenly turn on you and get physically aggressive. For example, she wouldn't let helpers get her fellow resident, Art, ready for bed—she thought he was her husband and the helpers were intruding. She would beat on Art's bedroom door until a helper opened it, then with a wild look in her eyes, flail out with her fists. When she had this look, helpers knew she was off in another reality and it was hard to reach her. It's not unusual for residents to think that one of the other residents is their husband or wife. Bonding like this can add a delicious sweetness to residents' lives, but sometimes, as in Olga's case, it can trigger aggression.

Though there were behavior challenges with Olga, staff was able to handle them. One thing they did was put a plastic safety cover on the doorknob so she couldn't come into Art's room at bedtime. Or they would try to redirect her before bedtime so that she and Art were separated earlier in the evening. Even with the challenges she presented, everyone adored her. They missed her when she moved on to a nursing home because of a lack of funding. The family wished her to be in the home setting, but what Medical Assistance was willing to pay would not cover the cost of her care.

When Olga first entered a nursing home, her confusion increased and her overall condition declined. Staff felt badly when they first visited her to see the changes that had occurred. They gave as much information as they could to the new staff about Olga's habits and cares. When a couple of the Rakhma staff members visited her a few months later, she had adjusted well. They felt the new staff had gotten to know her and appreciated her for who she was. They observed her chatting in lyrical, unintelligible syllables in her Scandinavian accent—"Ya, ya, ya" —with other residents. It appeared that she had bonded with some new friends. They were happily relieved; they could let the other helpers know Olga was all right.

More often, however, residents decline after they move and sometimes even die within a few months. I wonder if preconceived notions about nursing homes cause despondency, if another adjustment is just too much, or if, no matter how well-intentioned the nursing home staff is, there just isn't enough personal interaction to keep the resident connected in a meaningful way to the fabric of life.

Genevieve's Story

Genevieve is someone who falls through the cracks in the system. She needs assistance with baths and skin care for her psoriasis. She has dementia, but is still relatively independent. After being at Rakhma for three years, she depleted her personal funds. She would like to have stayed, but she couldn't get the funding she needed to pay for her nonmedical care at Rakhma.

Genevieve was the only Rakhma resident who left for an assisted living setting instead of a nursing home. She would have just enough social security and retirement money to pay for living there and she wanted to live as independently as she had at Rakhma. However, once she was on her own without supervision, she didn't take baths, didn't take care of her skin, and forgot her medications. Flaky skin in the air around her reminded visitors of Pigpen, the *Peanuts* comic strip character who was followed by a cloud of dust wherever he went. Other people wouldn't sit by her and she became more and more isolated. The manager of her assisted-living home expressed concern about the situation. Genevieve's conservator felt she would need to go to a nursing home to get the assistance and structure she needed. Her extra, nonmedical care would be paid for because nursing-home care is funded across the board, but what would be missing would be a sense of home.

Genevieve is just one real-life example of how regulatory inequities make it possible for nursing homes to get more reimbursement than a shared home for the kind of care she needs. As discussed in Chapter 4, this kind of regulatory inequity needs to be addressed across the country so that consumers are given options for their care regardless of ability to pay.

On a visit to Genevieve, we brought flowers. She had wet underpants that smelled of urine hanging on the radiator in her room. We brought her bakery cookies in a bag. She adores cookies of her own.

Steve Felsenberg, a former Minneapolis nursing home administrator now living in Boston, says that to make it financially, a home must have 100 to 150 residents. He laments, however, the dearth of life-enhancing care available when numbers are the game and the bottom line is the focus. The care becomes custodial only, management walks a tenuous regulatory tightrope, and nursing home residents, especially those without families (but those with families as well), face years of virtual warehousing. Though working with the elderly is Steve's chosen career, he left his position because he could no longer reconcile such barren care options with his personal integrity or his career goals.

We will look at the necessity for new paradigms of care in chapter 10, "Where Do We Go From Here?"

Families in Partnership

Rakhma is constantly working on ways to define how to best do its program and safeguard its residents. Where there are standard-size hallways instead of wide corridors, where there are chairs and tables placed in configurations that make a house a home, the reality with elderly residents is that there are going to be some bumps and falls.

When does minor tippiness cross the line to become major unsteadiness? How many falls are too many? How do you balance the need to keep people on their feet for muscle tone and fitness with the need to keep them safe? What about the decline in strength when a resident spends more and more time sitting during the day? If a resident sits in a recliner all day, how does staff and family handle the shift to total care that is inevitable as the person's muscle tone and strength decline?

Often staff does some pretty creative problem solving. One pacer kept bumping into things, putting herself at risk, and requiring constant supervision. Staff knew she loved the dining room best, so they closed it off at certain times and let her walk around the table to her heart's content. They could keep an eye on her and at the same time she could walk by herself in a safe place.

One woman with balance problems liked to walk barefoot. It seemed to make her feel better, so the staff allowed her to do it. At an Alzheimer's conference that year, Pam Boyce learned of a study by Ruth Tappen, Ed. D., R.N., from the school of nursing at the University of Miami, that showed walking barefoot for thirty minutes three times a week significantly improved communication in people with Alzheimer's disease. Dr. Tappen speculates that the exercise may stimulate part of the brain associated with handling communication. She stressed that the research, inspired by her own experience working with people with Alzheimer's, is still in its infancy, but is nonetheless promising.

This resident seemed to be more grounded when walking barefoot on the floor. To my way of thinking, it kept the soles of her feet in touch with reality. For Alzheimer's victims, having lost touch with a lot, the sensations of the feet touching the floor help maintain balance. And of course, walking barefoot massages the feet and strengthens the muscles.

When families understand Rakhma's dedication to care, even when a resident has to leave, it all works. Most families work closely with Rakhma staff, and whether or not their loved one stays or leaves for another setting, they have loving memories of the care their mom or dad received and the support available for the family.

Beverly moved in last fall from a town about forty miles away. She insisted on being on her feet all the time, walking constantly from room to room. When her brain said turn, her body would not listen, and plunk, down she would go. She moved faster than other people, pushed them along sometimes, often tripped over their feet. She had one fall after another and, in her constant moving, made the other residents more vulnerable to falling. The Rakhma staff and I called a care conference after one of the monthly potluck dinners. We let the family know that, though we loved Beverly's wonderful, dry sense of humor, we were concerned about her safety and could not care for her any longer in the home setting. Though the family wanted their mother to stay, they understood the risks and sprang into action to follow through on what was best for their mom and the other residents. In less than a week they found a residence closer to home, one of the places that Rakhma recommended to them that has very good Alzheimer's care. It was a case of a terrific working partnership with the family. They placed their mom in a more structured setting, but still a good one. All rejoiced.

However, there are situations where the family is bitter. They want their loved one to stay at Rakhma, no matter what. You do your work in the best faith, but it doesn't always have a happy ending. You don't want the family angry because you couldn't keep a loved one, but they sometimes don't understand the reality of the situation, and it leaves me with a sadness. I don't think they even understand why they are angry. It's a loss for them, a difficult time. The family may become silent and cut off. Or they make threats. Or they blame.

Even if a person can't stay with us, staff goes to the next setting to help pave the way. In the case of a bitter family, we still go the extra mile for the resident, not for thanks but to be true to our commitment to that person. And we bless the family with love and let them go. We don't want to hang on to that bitterness or sadness. We just let them go with love.

However, sometimes when a resident who left on unpleasant terms is dying, the family will take a new look at the time at Rakhma, make contact again, and see Rakhma's part in their life in a more charitable light.

Staying in Touch

Even having left on the best of terms, families often forget to stay in touch with Rakhma after their loved one leaves. They don't remember how much we cared for that person, or they don't realize how much like family each resident becomes. We really grow to care about each individual and want to know before we read in the paper of his or her funeral. We would like to know when someone who was once with us seems to be dying, even if it is a false alarm. People don't think about this, but why wouldn't we want to be there? To me it doesn't make sense not to be there and honor that person.

When early resident Hilda died, her family did not let Rakhma know. A year later, when I got word that Hilda was gone, Rakhma had a memorial service so staff who still remembered her could mark her passing. The family came and took part in the service.

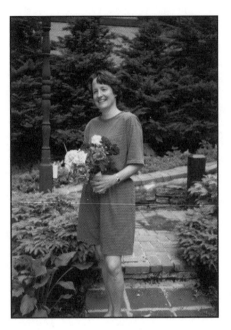

Colles Larkin

In Loving Memory

Sometimes the actual funeral service is held at Rakhma. Particularly when a resident has died in the home, the family wants the funeral service to be where the person has been living. A minister gathers relatives and friends in the intimacy of the Rakhma living room and conducts a simple, loving ceremony accompanied by piano and song.

"Rakhma is the one place I think that really makes an effort with Alzheimer's patients to give them their dignity," says Colles Larkin, whose mother Wilhelmina's funeral was held in the Grace living room. "When mother was there, one girl on her day off came in to hold mom's hand and talk to her when she was dying." The day she died, there were two or three in the room waiting with Willie until Colles could get there. "The sense of community is remarkable in the truest sense of the word," declares Colles.

Colles planned a memorial at Rakhma that also served as her mother's funeral service. A husband and wife musical duo plucked haunting melodies on the Irish harp in honor of Willie's Celtic heritage. Residents and staff joined the small gathering of relatives amid fresh flowers and trays of food.

The essence of the tiny, elegant woman with a ready smile that lit up the world filled the room. Through the readings, the songs, the ceremony, and particularly the sharing, the spirit of an educated woman, a wonderful mother, a sensitive human being lived.

"Love does not die with death," wrote Wilhelmina in a letter to Colles that was read at the memorial. "It endures to help enrich the lives of the living. As you well know, life is not trouble free, but, invariably, the clouds are overtaken by sunshine. And so often the artist who paints a clouded landscape paints with greater beauty and truth."

Colles had about a week to prepare for her mother's death. "It happened," her mother told her. Though Colles couldn't tell what had happened, it seemed to her that her mother had had a vision of some kind. She said, "Colles, I can't protect you anymore." At that moment Colles realized that even though she was in her fifties, her mother's comforting presence had always provided a kind of buffer. "I was learning from her up until the end," she remarked. During that last week, Willie reached out her hand. "I took her hand," said Colles, "but I saw later she was reaching beyond me."

When the funeral is held elsewhere, in most cases there is an additional memorial service in the house within two to three weeks. In case of sudden death, there are prayer services for the deceased. Even if the family doesn't wish to attend a memorial service, as a way of closure Rakhma still has one for the residents and staff who were not able to attend the funeral.

Most families want to attend the memorial. Rakhma staff likes to have the family there so that they can be duly appreciated for their love and energy as family members. Each family is different, and love manifests in many ways, seen and unseen, but at Rakhma, no matter what the dynamics, family members continue to be integral to the life of the resident and the home. I don't think we can ever appreciate families enough. They are welcome to come back any time.

Lynn's mother, Dorothy, died in the hospital with complications from a broken hip and pneumonia. Her Alzheimer's disease had brought her to Rakhma two years before.

On a cold day in January, house manager Winnie, resident Genevieve, and I all attended her funeral at Incarnation Catholic Church. Three weeks later a memorial was held at Peace Home where Dorothy had lived with such dignity the last two years of her life. Lynn's family helped prepare the service with the help of the Rakhma staff. Everyone in attendance got a packet that included a pen and ink sketch of Dorothy by Elizabeth Manfredi. The program went like this:

Opening Prayer . . . . .Winifred Tawo
Hymn . . . . .How Great Thou Art
Reading . . . . .Lynn Baskfield
Sharing Memories . . . . .All
Tape about Dorothy's Journey . . . . .Junice McCoy
Hymn . . . . .I Walk in the Garden Alone
Prayer of Peace . . . . .St. Francis of Assisi
Closing Words . . . . .Shirley Joy Shaw

Fellow resident Marcella had continually tried to get Dorothy to eat more at dinner and was forever concerned about how she picked at her food. Always the cultivated hostess, at the memorial she spoke eloquently and frequently about what a fine and gracious lady Dorothy had been, even though she didn't quite remember the details. As family, staff, and some of the residents shared about Dorothy's life, there was a sense of being enveloped in a great circle of love, of which Dorothy was still a part. Other residents joined in the singing. The reading went like this:

I am standing upon the seashore. A ship at my side spreads her white sails to the morning breeze and starts for the blue ocean. She is an object of beauty and strength. I stand and watch her until at length she hangs like a speck of white cloud just where the sea and sky come to mingle with each other.

Then someone at my side says: "There, she is gone!"

"Gone where?"

Gone from my sight. That is all. She is just as large in mast and hull and spar as she was when she left my side and she is just as able to bear her load of living freight to her destined port.

Her diminished size is in me, not in her. And just at the moment when someone at my side says: "There, she is gone!" there are other eyes watching her coming, and other voices ready to take up the glad shout: "Here she comes!"

And that is dying.

—Anonymous

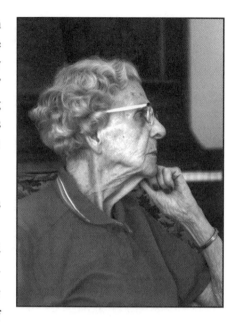

Dorothy Baskfield

Staff member Myrna, a gifted photographer, gave each of the family members an eight-by-ten copy of a color photo she had taken of Dorothy, her soft gray hair and pink blouse collar framing a thoughtful, faraway expression, the Rakhma piano in the background. Myrna had been especially close to Dorothy, patient and caring in the face of repetitive questions about where she would stay and how she would get to breakfast in the morning. She was the only helper Dorothy always remembered and she shared, in her gentle way, about the special times they had spent together before bed at the end of each day.

"The memorial was nice," reflected granddaughter Shannon, "because it showed the family that Grandma was really cared about. It was individual. Intimate. It showed me that in that home the resident is a person, a member of a family, not just a client that pays the bills. You don't find that very many places and I'm glad my Grandma got to be a part of that."

Dying at Home: Hospice at Rakhma

Not to be confused with the hospice movement where special homes are set up for people with incurable illnesses, hospice at Rakhma has to do with

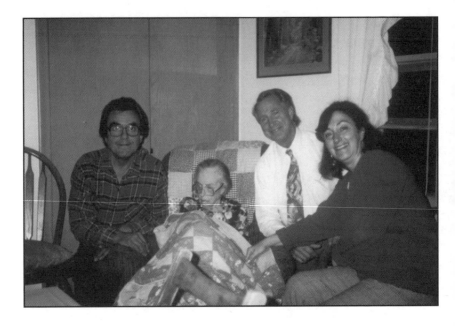

Helen B. and family

the natural progression of being with a resident through the time of dying.
Perhaps the resident is not eating or wants to sleep all the time. The doctor
says there's nothing that can be fixed; the person is just closing down. There
is a reframing. It's a case of giving comfort and love rather than longer life.
The family, at that point, doesn't want to move them from our setting.

We do hospice with agreement from the resident's doctor, the Rakhma
staff, and family members. If the person needs nurse supervision, which happens only occasionally, we have the family call in an outside nurse. But mostly
it's about loving comfort. The family can be there most of the time, as much
as they want to. We see to it that there is nice soft music, the kind the dying
resident likes, and something pretty to look at when they open their eyes.

At hospice time, you have to get staff to understand that the family and
the resident has requested this. By now there is a DNR/DNI order in place,
so there will be no measures taken to prolong life. Even though in our line

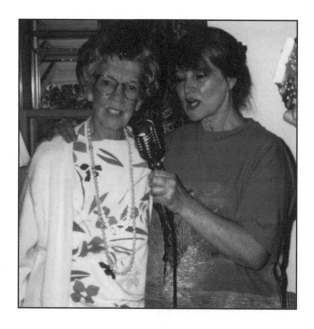

Helen Lund singing with Myrna

of work we expect that people will die eventually, staff has loved that resident and doesn't always understand why they have to go. Our part is to honor their time of leaving. Once the staff understands this they work pretty well with it, but it's hard to let go.

Kitty Smith, a dear friend of mine and the "mother of hospice" in Minnesota, reminded staff at an in-service she conducted shortly before her own death what an honor it is to be with people when they are dying. It's almost like being with someone when they are being born, she observed. Each one leaves in his or her own way. Some are very peaceful in taking their last breath. Some want to sit up and be part of everyday life until their head goes to the side and they are gone.

Kitty's in-service piqued staff member Myrna's interest in hospice work, which she now does in addition to her regular shifts. A very gentle, loving helper, she provides a special touch that families ask for during their

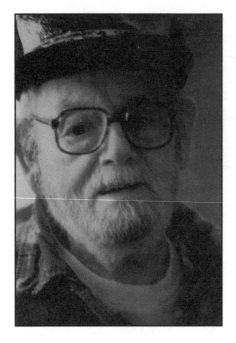

Ernest Meili

loved one's hospice time. Myrna even comes in at night to be with dying residents. Her presence is a rare gift.

When Ernest "Grandpa" Meili could no longer walk the stairs to his second-floor bedroom, staff moved him into the sunroom on the main floor of Rakhma Home 1. He had been doing poorly. When his daughter took him to the doctor to see what was wrong, the doctor simply said, "There isn't anything to do. It's time for Mr. Meili to say good-bye."

Grandpa had always loved being out of doors. Now Rakhma helpers kept the sunroom windows open so he could see the trees outside through lace curtains that blew in the summer breezes Though he didn't want to eat, Mr. Meili would take little sips of water. For a while he talked philosophically about God, but as the days passed he spoke less and less. Seini, the house manager at the time, sat with him one day toward the end, massaging his scalp. "I love you" he said softly into the silence.

The next day Ernest's breathing became harder. His family, who had come to be with him, drew the curtain across the sunroom archway and stayed at his side for a very long time. When his daughter finally emerged from his room, she spoke through tears of loss and tears of joy. "It's so nice that Dad could die here with the sun coming in and the flowers in the window boxes. He loved being outside so much. It felt so right that he could be right here."

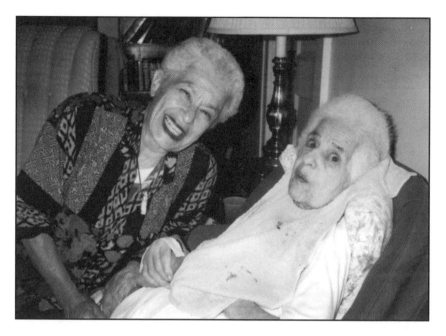

Sally Flax and Mom, Queen Isabelle of Rakhma

To Keep in Mind...

- The Rakhma model keeps residents with behavior problems a little longer than other settings might in order to creatively assimilate the person into the household if possible.

- Ongoing assessment of each resident makes it possible to respond to their real needs.

- There is follow up when a resident moves on to another setting:
  —With the staff at the new setting.
  —With the resident.
  —With the resident's family.

- Staff members and residents who are able attend the funerals of residents who die.

- There is an in-house memorial service for each resident to:
  —Allow staff and residents to feel complete.
  —Acknowledge family.

- Being with a resident in the home setting at the time of dying is a natural progression of care. This way of honoring a resident's leaving may be set up at the request of family, with medical permission.

CHAPTER 9

They Return It in a Thousand Ways
Volunteers

To the question, "How can I help?" we now see the possibility of a deeper answer than we might once have expected. We can, of course, help through all that we do. But at the deepest level we help through who we are.

> —Ram Das and Paul Gorman,
> *How Can I Help? Stories and Reflections on Service*

I love it! What a joy to just do something for someone else who can't return the favor. But they do! They return it in a thousand ways, just by BEING; by responding to my smile, and allowing me to be myself. I receive much more from them than anyone could ever repay with gratuities.

> —Nona Hanson, Rakhma Volunteer

The daily demands of a shared home stared me square in the eye. I quickly saw that even with a good staff in place, I couldn't do everything that still needed to be done and be everywhere that people wanted me to be. Although there was no coordinated volunteer program until 1989, volunteers began early on to help with the many needs of the fledgling organization. As I mentioned earlier, Lynn's sister Barbara came to Rakhma 1 once a week, made cookies, created lovely meals, and took people for walks. Lynn did development work, public relations outreach, proposal writing, and budget projections. Mary Dobbins gave legal advice; board member Gloria Feik, real estate expertise; and board member Mary Ondov, all encompassing strength and wisdom. Others filled in with donations, visits, ideas, repair work, and music. A volunteer program evolved as Rakhma evolved.

My long-time friend and canoeing pal, Pam Boyce, was vice president of an estate-sale company. She had volunteered at Rakhma since it first opened, finding treasures for the Rakhma homes through her sales. After six years of working for the estate-sale company, Pam decided it was time for a change in her career. I asked her if she would consider working at Rakhma as a volunteer coordinator. Pam joined the Rakhma staff on a trial basis as the third house was about to open. She took a pay cut and did an estate sale each month for a while for extra income, but soon found that her new work was perfect—she loved people, wanted the challenge of developing a role for herself in the organization, and was self-motivated. As she looked at existing volunteers and activities, she felt that the residents needed to have more happening in their lives with more outside energy. Her goal: to recruit more volunteers and plan activities to enhance the lives of residents and volunteers alike.

It takes a special person to volunteer with residents who have Alzheimer's disease, one who can esteem the resident whether or not he or she is suddenly losing interest in the activity at hand, or is having behavior problems that day. Residents are changeable. Volunteers who stay with us have to get past the discomfort of seeing this happen. In a twinkling of an eye a resident can be interested in doing a craft or an art project, and then not want to do it at all.

Volunteering at Rakhma is about whatever it is that day. You are there to be present and help bring the residents joy. It might not be visibly rewarding. It may feel like you're not making a difference sometimes. Some days there is no thanks from the residents. We remind our caregivers to be sensitive to that, so that they can let our volunteers know they are appreciated even if the residents can't.

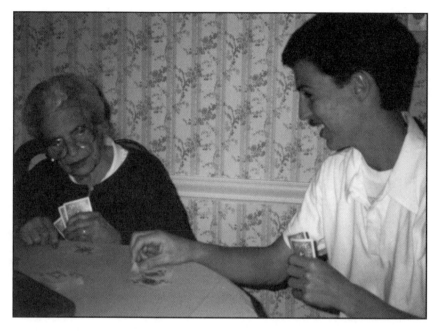

Hilda playing cards with student from Academy of the Holy Angels

Pam has made it a point to nurture her volunteers in many small ways. First of all, volunteers are given an orientation about Rakhma and a profile of the residents that specifies what they like and don't like. For instance, one loves to read, one may enjoy dancing, and another delights in going for a walk. One may not like to be asked direct questions about her past because it upsets her that she can't remember the answers. Others like to be hugged or have their hands held. Pam talks about the importance of touch and how it's not always easy to see that you make a difference as a volunteer. She assures them that they do, that without them, Rakhma can't survive; the residents thrive on the attention volunteers provide. Then volunteers are given time to learn about the residents by observing them.

Pam always makes sure the volunteers feel appreciated by doing things like sending them thank you notes, giving them photos taken during activities which included them, featuring a volunteer in the *Rakhma Heartbeat* newsletter, having a volunteer appreciation week, and just loving them as if they were members of her own family.

Pam says that volunteers are like fresh air—they bring in new faces and new activities to the homes. When residents get belligerent, it's usually with the staff who are trying to direct them in their daily cares. Because volunteers don't work as caregivers, they are more likely to be perceived as welcome friends coming to visit.

Pam has developed an outreach network that helps make and maintain volunteer connections. She goes to functions sponsored by volunteer placement organizations, meets their staff, and invites staff from those organizations to the Rakhma homes. She finds the personal contact to be invaluable. One volunteer placement worker, since getting to know Pam and the Rakhma Homes, now sends volunteers regularly. The simple act of being related opened the door.

A local high school sends students to volunteer each year. A group of singing corporate retirees, the Honeybelles, are part of Pam's network. Announcements for volunteer openings in the city and neighborhood papers bring good response. There are connections with Macalester College in the Joy Home neighborhood. Churches send lay ministers and visitors who give one-on-one time to residents or bring communion. Pam acknowledges that when she starts thinking about needing volunteers, something begins to happen. The outreach structure is important, but there is an unknown force, she says, "that once you start paying attention and tap into it—we need more volunteers now—it gets flowing again. It's an interesting balance to keep. We need to keep the channels open."

Through the Eyes of Volunteers

In any organization, volunteering is a two-way street. It must meet the needs of the organization as well as the needs of the volunteer. Each party comes away having been enriched, having learned something, and having made

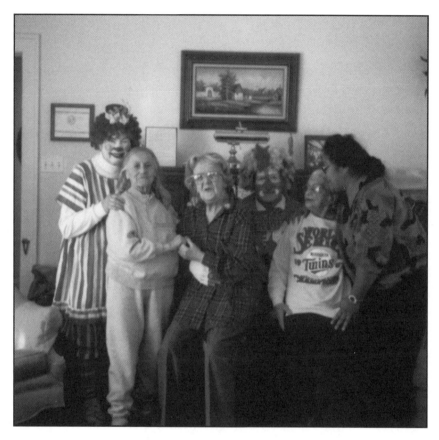

Honeybelle clowns at Rakhma Peace Home

a difference. Volunteers at Rakhma range in age from high school students to retirees.

Jenny Brav was a student coordinator of a senior citizens program on the Macalester College campus, where she was taking courses in adult aging and development. Rakhma was one of the establishments with which her program worked regularly, and it had piqued her curiosity because, located only a few blocks from campus, it was a home that looked very much like the other stately homes on Wheeler Street, not at all institutional like the other nursing homes she worked with. In addition, its neighborhood parties created a cohesiveness and awareness of the surrounding environment, which Jenny and her coworkers felt to be very important. She decided to do a site visit partly out of curiosity and partly because she had never been in contact with Alzheimer's patients before and wanted to know more about the disease. After the site visit, she decided to volunteer for two reasons: she had never worked in a home setting before, and she wanted to test her bias that people with Alzheimer's disease had very little ability to communicate and process information. She hoped to prove her bias wrong. Her work at Rakhma enhanced her academic studies as well and became the foundation of an insightful paper on Alzheimer's disease.

Nona Hanson's quote at the beginning of this chapter showcases her irrepressible spirit. The daughter of a preacher and a devoted mom who ministered to the needs of their parish during the Depression, she grew up to understand that everyone has an influence on someone else, and each person can make this world a better place even in small ways, every day.

Hers has been a life of active service—to her family, friends, church, and those in need. Although she has now retired from full-time nursing, she has not retired from life. She remains active as a substitute nurse in the schools and works with the free clinic at her church.

"Ah, Pam," she says, "bless her for placing the ad in the local paper stating the need for a piano player for a senior residence. The ad jumped out as if it were meant just for me. I have always loved to play the piano, though without formal training, it's mostly by ear. I began playing for church when I was only nine, as I was the only one available. People have always encouraged me by allowing me to be less than perfect.

"I'm still not perfect! Surprised? I must continually practice those old songs and change the keys to accommodate our voices and work on those accidentals which seem to crop up in the simplest of songs. But the girls at Rakhma Home put up with me and they sing their hearts out. It's such fun to hear them sing the old songs and remember the words when many of them have current memory lapses. They often request the same songs over and over on the same day, which is great as long as they participate and enjoy themselves. They especially like the motion songs, such as 'Deep and Wide' and 'Alleluia, Praise Ye the Lord.' The boys from the Academy of the Holy Angels Religious Education Class bring life and enthusiasm with them that makes for a great day.

Volunteers from all walks of life come to Rakhma to help others, to share the gifts they have been given, to add structure to their day, or simply because they read about the volunteer opportunities at Rakhma and it seems to be a fit.

Some choose Rakhma for convenience—it is close to home. Others like it because it is a smaller facility. Others hear positive things about Rakhma or can work out a flexible time frame for helping out. One of the volunteer musicians chose it because she believes music can touch the souls of any age, and another came because her sister volunteered there. She felt she could help not only the residents but her sister too.

Some have had Alzheimer's disease strike a family member and want to understand more about it. One mom with small children wants them to be around older people. Another woman's grandmother lives far away and misses being with older people herself. Often people volunteer who have, through a variety of circumstances, come to understand how fortunate they are and wish to be of service to others.

Even having heard positive things about Rakhma, many of the volunteers are pleasantly surprised the first day they arrive, as was Nona. "My first visit to Rakhma was a surprise," she said, "because I thought I would see the usual dormitory style of a care facility which is so common these days. However, to my delight, this home is in an older, established neighborhood, an area where I would love to live. I was warmly greeted by Pam, who took me on a tour of the home, which smelled wonderful. There always seems to be something cooking, and there were flowers on the dining-room table, over which hangs a lovely chandelier. Flowers also brightened up the tastefully furnished living room, which contained lovely, overstuffed furniture and an old upright piano that made the place seem so friendly and homey. The sunshine streamed through the lace-curtained windows and the ladies smiled at me and appeared to be very contented, as if they had arrived for a lovely luncheon. Also present was a cute little toddler who enjoyed being patted and a little poodle who seemed to need special care in its senior years as well. What a privilege to be able to enjoy the fellowship of these wonderful people."

Jenny Brav reports that Pam told her the only prerequisites for volunteering were caring and being self-motivated. She warned her that there wouldn't be much structure to the volunteer experience, and that she would have to decide for herself what she wanted to do. This might range from simply sitting with one resident and holding her hand to organizing a chair aerobics session with a group of residents. In the beginning, Jenny felt frustrated at what looked like lack of organization, "but I realized after a while that, in fact, the backbone of their days, such as meals, outings, etc., was very structured, but within that framework the staff members were flexible. I do believe that, considering the situation of the residents, a group home is probably one of the best settings for people with Alzheimer's disease, and much more humane than some of the Alzheimer's wards I have seen in nursing homes."

Things that volunteers often mention when asked what they enjoy most about being at Rakhma is the uniqueness of the environment, the loving atmosphere, the sense of family among staff, residents, and residents' family members, the smiles on the residents' faces and the smiles they bring. Retired CPA Tom Muehlbruer, now a volunteer pianist, tells of a Rakhma resident who asked him if he was a music teacher by profession. Tom had to say, "No, I'm an accountant."

The resident's response: "Why would a nice guy like you want to be an accountant?" This tickled Tom's funny bone, and he took the rejoinder as a compliment of the highest order.

A Uniquely Personal Experience
Volunteering is a uniquely personal experience, and each person gleans different rewards from time spent in service to others. In almost every case, when the volunteer experience is a fit and a volunteer stays at Rakhma for a period of time, he or she reports coming away with unexpected insights.

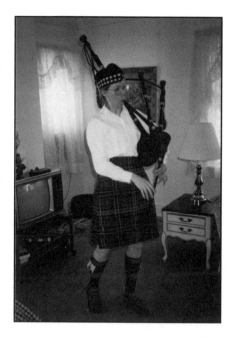

The realization that Alzheimer's disease can strike anyone is sobering. It is an all-too-real reminder that the volunteer may need the kind of services someday that they are now providing. That many people who were highly intelligent can be thus afflicted in

Nancy Wilson playing the bagpipes

their later years can be depressing sometimes, but also, according to one volunteer, "I am reminded that life is too short to permit insignificant things to be an issue. I have learned from my experience to enjoy each day and each person fully."

Another volunteer was pleasantly surprised to find that the people at Rakhma were lovable, loving, and responsive, had their unique personalities, and really cared about one another.

Jenny has thought about this, too: "One thing which I found very interesting was that, even with the disease, the residents still maintained their own distinct personalities. I think many people think of Alzheimer's patients, especially those in the advanced stages of the disease, as being devoid of memory, logical speech patterns, and most other distinguishing characteristics. One woman did suffer from a definite memory loss, and two of the women did not speak at all. However, among those who did, there were recurrent patterns to their conversations, actions, etc. Alice, for example, has a granddaughter at Macalester, and even though one week it would be her grandson, the next her nephew, and the next her son, she always remembered having a relative going there.

"Alice is a socialite, and every time I see her she is waiting to go somewhere. She is usually cheerful and smiling, and she always pronounces everything to be wonderful. The way she has coped with the disease is by creating her own world, which is probably fuller and more beautiful than many people's real lives. The other day it was a dark, dreary and snowy day, and she looked out the window and said to me, 'Isn't it a nice day? All that sun.'

"I have given her numerous back rubs, which she always appreciates tremendously and never wants to end. She loves being with people. She always referred to another resident, Ceil, as her friend. When Ceil had to leave to go to another home, I was worried about Alice. However, the next time I went to Rakhma Joy, she was sitting next to Norma and holding her hand. Norma doesn't talk, which is why I didn't expect her to be the one to replace Ceil. She mostly sits on the couch and sleeps and drools, but Alice likes being with her. I think it's beautiful, because I expected the residents in the early stages to group together, but Alice just cares for everyone indiscriminately. Last time I was there she sat down between Norma and me and she said of Norma, 'Poor girl, she's having a hard time, you know.'"

One volunteer mentioned that she learned that much can be accomplished in helping Alzheimer's patients through love and concern. Another has cultivated a great respect and gratitude for old age; being in the prayers of the residents moves her. Yet another finds herself unsure that she is getting through to the residents. "I know in my heart," she says, "that many times they have been touched but simply do not display it."

Jenny looks at it this way: Being part of many nonsensical conversations with Rakhma residents, she realized how culturally important verbal communication is, as well as how void it can be. She became more aware of what she calls her buffer sentences, generic phrases to fit any situation. Working with Alzheimer's patients demanded less reliance on verbal communication and brought about for her a new awareness of her tone of voice and facial expressions, aspects of communication to which Alzheimer's patients are very sensitive.

"I rid my speech pattern of superfluous terms and abstract concepts, returning to the basic nature of communication. It was interesting how oral communication became secondary, and words were only used as reassurance or to convey a direct and simple message. I fell into a pattern of repeating the same thing as many times as necessary, until it became so automatic I paid much more attention to the other senses such as touch. I gave many back and hand massages."

The volunteers who bring music communicate with the music. People in all stages of life, mental ability, and comprehension enjoy music. Said one, "I love to play music, especially waltzes and polkas, and I love to see people keeping time with the music with their hands and feet." Said another, "It is beautiful to see the reactions of the people listening."

Volunteers, from coordinator Pam's point of view as mentioned earlier, are like fresh air for the residents, bringing friendship and a sense of normalcy with their visits. One volunteer, Carol Preston, even goes to the quarterly potluck dinners so she can meet the families of the residents she works with and place them in the larger context of the community they came from.

A Little Distance

While volunteers often become close to the residents, because they are not family members who have a history with the person when they were well, there is a certain distance. A volunteer can relate to the residents in their dementia in a way that family members cannot. Catherine, when her daughter was visiting, would say over and over, "Today is today. Today is today is today." Her daughter would keep agreeing, but I could tell she was having trouble seeing her mother in that state and had to fight back exasperation. It made me wonder how I would react if it were my own mother in the home, and that was tough for me to think about.

It is tough, but some who have a relative at Rakhma volunteer there also and find it quite workable. The pleasant, safe, family-like environment is conducive to learning how to be with a loved one and with others who have memory loss. You do not have to figure it out alone. There is strength in numbers, and being in an environment that accepts that "funny" behavior gives the family member a larger framework in which to hold the changes their loved one has experienced.

Hilda's granddaughter Krista started as a volunteer at Rakhma when she was about twelve years old so she could spend more time with her grandmother. At age sixteen, she became a certified nursing assistant and worked from then through college at the home her grandmother lived in. She was a loving, sensitive helper. Dorothy's grandson was the Rakhma Peace Santa Claus for a couple of years. Her daughter Barbara is now on the board of directors, having gained a great deal of understanding about Alzheimer's disease from her experience with her mother and having learned a great deal about Rakhma, its philosophy and model of care, while her mother was there. Many others have filled volunteer niches at Rakhma, enriched and motivated by the support they received there as family members confronted with an unpredictable and incurable disease.

Bill, a volunteer of two years, was stricken with AIDS. Having worked with Alzheimer's disease, he had a special understanding of what people went through with a progressive, incurable illness. Pam was one of the first to know about his condition, and felt it important that the staff should be educated about AIDS. Even though Bill decided to take care of himself and withdraw from his volunteer activities, the local AIDS association provided educational materials and a speaker who did an in-service for the Rakhma staff.

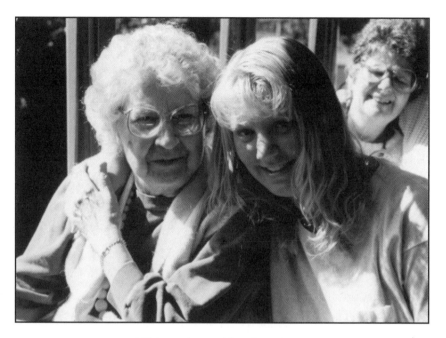

Hilda and granddaughter Krista

Bill and Pam had developed a close friendship, staying in touch by phone and then by mail when he moved out of state to spend his final days with family. Before he left, he came to say good-bye. He wanted Rakhma to have some of his furniture. Bill was a loving and spiritual person who had found a special peace.

Volunteering at Rakhma has a way of drawing people into life. With Bill, his sense of service was heightened there in the face of his own mortality. With others, it's perhaps not so poignantly tenuous as facing one's own death, but it draws forth, nevertheless, an awareness of the interconnectedness of life, the unpredictability and joy contained therein. Volunteer Carol Preston observed, "I taught music for a few years and now it is fun to play all the oldies but goodies. If my former students could hear the nonclassical music I am playing on the keyboard, it would surprise them. One of the residents referred to my renditions as ballroom music. This was a real compliment for me, as my father played in a small band for dances for many years. I envision him in the Great Beyond, winking at me and saying, 'I knew you could do it.' "

Challenges

Although for the most part, being a volunteer at Rakhma has its rewards, there are challenges, too. One volunteer finds that staying innovative and bringing new ideas for activities is much harder than just doing the same old things every week. Several have mentioned that being confronted with the possibility of getting Alzheimer's disease someday themselves is frightening. Jenny sometimes feels anger when she sees residents who were once active and involved drooling on themselves. She and others feel frustrated by the lack of scientific knowledge we have about the disease and the inability to be of real help to those who suffer from it. Finding time to keep coming back is an issue for busy volunteers, although most make it a priority despite schedule crunches.

Occasionally there are sticky situations brought about by a resident's behavior. For example, the residents love Doug, a volunteer in his thirties who comes to read aloud and share conversation. One of the residents, however, has lost her inhibitions as her Alzheimer's has progressed and likes to tease him and pinch him on the behind. When Doug is there, she says inappropriate things to him and embarrasses him. He doesn't really know what to do, so he gets up and walks out of the room.

As with any difficulty like this, Pam works on ways to solve the problem. We don't want to lose volunteers. We want it to be the best experience for the volunteer, yet not take away the dignity of the resident. These are some approaches Pam has taken to alleviate the problem.

- Doug comes weekly. When he arrives staff see if they can get the resident involved in the kitchen area cutting veggies, or occupy her with something else.

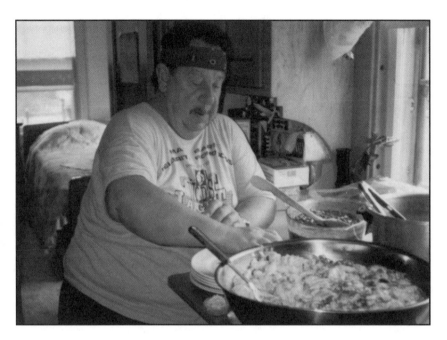

Curt Carlson, volunteer cook

- If the resident is inappropriate, catch it right away, take her out of the room and speak to her. Behavior modification may work with some residents.

- Orient volunteers to each person's behavior. For example, explain to Doug situationally about this resident's behavior.

- Take the resident out of the house for a walk or for an outing when a particular volunteer comes.

Getting to know the residents is crucial. When we've had a volunteer for a while, they get to know the residents and eventually find a comfortable niche for themselves. It often takes some flexibility. Musicians come who think they will concentrate on playing music, but find that residents enjoy singing. They wind up not just playing music, but singing and maybe even dancing as well. A retired teacher brings gifts of stimulation and color through crafts and planned activities, but sometimes finds that talking about spring or picking a basket of flowers is what is needed that day. A volunteer cook not only adds great new recipes to Wednesday lunches, but after being at Rakhma a while, asks if he can cozy up the kitchen. Objects he brings catch the light from the south window and the kitchen, thanks to him, is a warmer, friendlier place to be.

Other challenges cited by volunteers are that Rakhma needs more visibility in the community, that communication between the homes sometimes breaks down, and that the Volunteer Coordinator cannot be in all three homes at once.

One gift the volunteers bring is a broad view combined with a well-developed social consciousness. Several see themselves as part of a bigger whole, part of the solution, with something to give even in the midst of busy lives. A few like Jenny map their work at Rakhma onto an even broader conceptual framework. "My main critique," said Jenny, "would be a criticism of social policy concerning the lack of governmental aid which is provided to group homes. This is the reason that Ceil had to leave: her family could no longer afford it, even though Rakhma offers as much financial support as they can to residents who need it." Despite challenges, one volunteer is amazed that there is so little staff turnover. She feels this speaks well of the administration. Another appreciates the fact that the homes are run by very loving and caring people. "From what I have seen," she said, Rakhma is a very warm, friendly, clean home."

"May God bless you," says another, "for what you are doing for the elderly. It is the highest act of love." And so it is with the volunteers, too. The highest acts of love come grandly as merry music, joyfully as peals of laughter, or unobtrusively as a quiet conversation or the daily feeding of a resident at the evening meal, then sitting with her for a while after dinner. The volunteers are, indeed, a breath of fresh air, committed souls who come with an abundance of gifts to share, yet leave not depleted, but replenished.

As Nona's pastor, Larry LePoidiven, says, "Have you ever prayed for God to use you? People who pray for the Lord to use them, get used!"

To Keep in Mind...

- The requirements for being a volunteer in a home like Rakhma are two: a caring heart and self-motivation.

- Volunteers are oriented to the house in which they will work and to each person's behavioral characteristics.

- For the volunteer experience to work, the volunteer must get at least as much out of it as the residents or the organization does.

- Although a small home may look to the volunteer as if it is not organized, there is an overall structure that makes it possible to respond spontaneously to the daily needs of the residents.

- Residents with Alzheimer's disease forget, their attention lapses. and their moods change frequently, sometimes leaving the volunteer wondering if they are making a difference. Frequent acknowledgment of volunteers by administrative and caregiving staff is essential.

- Volunteers learn the value of touch, music, and other nonverbal forms of communication while working with people with dementia.

- Sometimes residents, in their disease, are inappropriate with volunteers. Rakhma's policy is to make the volunteer experience the best it can be for the volunteer while at the same time preserve the dignity of the resident.

CHAPTER 10

Where Do We Go From Here?

A graceful future is one open to psychological, political, and onto-
logical novelty. It emerges naturally from a life-style which centers in awareness of the vibrant present. Such openness is properly
called "Hope."

—Sam Keen, *To a Dancing God*

Three shared homes have been opened in the fourteen years since
Rakhma first began. Still, to find a home like Rakhma for an elderly
family member is not easy. So many people want non-nursing home care
that enables their loved ones to live out their years with dignity and love,
but hardly anything like that exists.

This chapter defines a vision for the future that includes making the
Rakhma model available to other communities around the nation. It includes
thoughts on educating families, schools, churches, and the community about
the privilege it is to have elderly family members, to share with them, and
to care for them. Making changes in legislation is another vital step that
must be taken, so that the shared-home category, the preferred setting for
so many, can receive funding that makes sense. There is no question that
more of these homes could be developed with the enlightened cooperation
of government and private-sector funders, as well as volunteer organizations. Even more importantly, this chapter is a call for a fundamental shift
in thinking, a new paradigm for elder care which transfers the emphasis
from governmentally imposed regulation to consumer-based contracts that

would allow for a much broader range of care options and provide a higher quality of life.

Where we go from here is really what Rakhma has been about all along: learning again and again about going the extra mile—and bringing that commitment to the elderly each new day.

Twenty Years Down the Road

Jonathan M. Evans, a Mayo Clinic geriatric physician practicing through the Community Internal Medicine Clinic in Rochester, Minnesota, grew up around grandparents who were an important part of his life. He went into medicine because he was drawn to people and felt that healing the sick was an important thing to do in one's life. He went into geriatrics because, through the influence of his grandparents, he was attracted to revering and honoring age.

As he pondered his career choice, Dr. Evans asked himself, "Do I have the qualities a doctor needs? Will I be able to connect with people on a very intimate level?" Those were the big questions for him, not "Can I make a comfortable living?" or "Will I be able to stay up at night?"

"If I were at the beach," smiles Dr. Evans, "I would spend the whole time finding shells and picking up rocks. I delight in finding things of value and beauty that are overlooked by other people. Geriatrics, there's where the disease is. It's an overlooked area, often frustrating to others because it's complicated. It entails multiple diseases coupled with multiple medications. It requires lots of detective work. For that very reason, I find it more fun."

Dr. Evans notes that as the population ages, there will be more and more people with Alzheimer's disease. Given a health-care system that is not equipped to handle all who need care now, he questions what is going to happen twenty years down the road. Nursing homes are filled with residents who have Alzheimer's disease or related disorders but who don't need the skilled care nursing homes were designed to provide. This situation impacts everyone because it creates a shortage of space for those who do need skilled care and is a wrong fit for those who don't.

Nursing homes are the hospitals of yesterday, according to Dr. Evans. Often elderly people are sent to a nursing home instead of going to a hospital for maladies ranging from pneumonia to anxiety to recovering from surgery. Nursing home care is based on a medical model: finding a cure within the context of health-care delivery. Nursing homes, by their very nature, are equipped to provide medical care to all who stay in them, including people with Alzheimer's disease and dementia.

"The world of people with Alzheimer's disease is different," comments Dr. Evans. Though labeled a disease, on the level of daily care it can't be treated as something to be cured. It does not require a technological approach. Rather, treating someone with Alzheimer's disease is a quality-of-life issue that must be addressed by getting into the world of the patient and making it a comfortable place to be.

People with Alzheimer's disease don't tolerate changes very well, says Dr. Evans. For instance, a doctor's office is not an ideal place for someone with memory loss. They get frustrated sitting in the lobby, may get agitated and leave upset. When they go to the hospital, there is even more confusion. Often they don't even know they are in the hospital. Restraints and medications are used to handle the agitation, putting the patient at risk of developing other problems.

"Nursing homes were never designed for this patient population," Dr. Evans emphasizes. "They were built on a hospital model. For someone who's confused and wandering, the environment could be dangerous. The whole system of health care was designed for conditions other than Alzheimer's disease. It's a risky place, to say nothing of quality-of-life issues that arise there."

What is needed is a paradigm shift, allowing people with Alzheimer's disease to live in a home environment, not an environment of skilled-care services that only someone with advanced training can provide. Caring for people with dementia requires separate specialized training focused on quality of life. "We would shift from a medical model to a quality-of-life model," he says.

Disease manifests itself differently in elderly people than in the general population. Very often, nonspecific symptoms bring elderly people to get medical attention. With Alzheimer's disease you might not be able to remember if you had chest pain, or other symptoms. Diagnosis requires sleuthing.

"Although a number of people want medicine to be a fountain of preservation, we focus on people doing more with what they have. We don't restrict ourselves to people living long; we want them to live well," says Dr. Evans. "We end up stopping more meds than starting them. When we ask what is the ideal environment for people with Alzheimer's disease to live in, we not only look at the more clinical aspects of physical health, unsteadiness, and what would promote independence yet decrease risk of serious injury from falling, but we look at two other aspects as equally important: human dignity and quality of life."

Remember House Calls?

Another model shift would be to provide care by seeing Alzheimer's patients at home. Dr. Evans makes a practice of going out to homes to see how patients are, often on his own time in the evening. He also works on the premises in a Kensington Cottage home, similar to Rakhma, in the area.

"Many of us feel a strong bond to community," he says, "and to patients as an extension of family. That's what we went into medicine for. What I do doesn't rely so much on technology as what the cardiologist does. The home environment has a lot of relevance for the patient. I can really tell how they thrive in their home environment. That's what geriatrics is all about. All physicians take care of the elderly, but that's why geriatrics is a specialty. With geriatrics how one is able to function in their environment is more important than the disease."

Dr. Evans feels it is hypocritical to tell elderly people how to live. "They can tell *me* how to live," he says. "In a culture that idolizes youth, there's a richness there that might escape me. On the other hand, people who are old have made it through something very difficult—life."

Education

I'd like there to be a lot more options for people with memory loss to feel connected. I'd like to make it possible for the old to share their creativity and their wisdom with the young. Educational avenues are many. The classroom is a good place to start.

At this point, Rakhma works with high schools and colleges providing volunteer opportunities that teach about the needs of the elderly and the richness that being with older people provides. In some cases, young volunteers choose careers in gerontology from their experience at Rakhma.

College-level gerontology classes visit Rakhma homes to look at alternative housing. However, these visits not only model the home, but they provide social awareness and inspire students to dream.

"I think my time at Rakhma has given me an important perspective that I will take with me through medical school and my practice as a physician," asserted Molly Benhin, after doing a month-long internship at the Joy Home. "This perspective involves the recognition of each patient as an individual. I have read so much about the pathophysiology of Alzheimer's disease and the typical profile of symptoms that it would be easy to see the residents as textbook cases. However, I have gotten to know each resident very intimately and I have a feel for her likes, dislikes, abilities, etc. I know that each resident's experiences with this memory disease are unique, so logically, different treatments and strategies are appropriate for each resident. I think that the way doctors are trained in our culture emphasizes the placing of patients in the category of a specific disorder, and this automatically dehumanizes each patient. I hope as a doctor, I can successfully mesh the traditional diagnostic processes of medicine with a true appreciation for each patient's uniqueness."

After spending some volunteer time at a very reputable, traditional nursing home, Molly said that by comparison, Rakhma is an ideal setup. She was impressed by the "humane, stimulating, loving environment" at Rakhma, and thinks that the Rakhma model could easily be applied to other kinds of facilities as the demand for alternative care grows with the growing population of seniors.

The Honored Elder

Rakhma revives the almost extinct tradition of the honored elder. The students who visit or volunteer are introduced to the residents as guests of the home. It is the residents who have the honored place, and even within the Rakhma household, the eldest resident is the respected elder. People rise to that honor, and why shouldn't they? Few of them have experienced an environment where the elderly are held in respect, particularly those elderly who are least "with it" mentally. Visiting Rakhma gives a glimpse of a possibility that hasn't been part of our experience, yet when students are exposed to it, it resonates: *Yes. How beautiful. Of course this is the natural order of life. This is what it looks like to honor our elders.*

And always I tell students that, if they can dream, they can do it. Whatever their vision is, pursue it. Most of the college students are going to be working with the elderly in some way, whether as social workers, administrators, doctors, or nurses. Seeing Rakhma inspires students to look at whatever track they might be on in a new way. Often they leave looking at themselves in a new way, too.

Our vision for the future includes educational outreach in the classroom at the grade and high-school levels teaching about the elderly. Unlike Dr. Evans, some kids don't even know their own grandparents. However, they could learn about their relationship to older people in school. Sometimes school curricula talk about how other cultures honor their elders. What about ours?

One way to implement this kind of training would be to design a series of teaching modules that senior volunteers could share in the classroom. (Junior Achievement does something like this now, teaching business principles with predesigned materials packets taught by volunteer businessmen and businesswomen.) Each module would include materials that

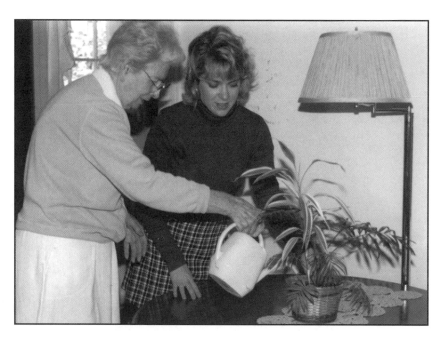

Resident Dorothy and Laurel, Assistant Director

illustrate the lesson, the most important thing being that each lesson provide a structure to allow the senior volunteer to share about his or her own life in a way that makes issues of aging very personal and very understandable. I call it "planting the seeds." It is important for children to know that elderly people started off as babies just like they did. It is important for children to hear the stories of the elders, to know of joy and sadness and the continuum of life. It is important to know that their hugs are needed by older people, that the elderly are special people, and that maybe they could bring flowers to an elderly neighbor or even ask their parents if they can invite that neighbor to their home.

Education must affect us personally. We can then make an impact in our homes and families as well as go beyond our own group and affect the larger community.

Community

According to Cheryl Biel, Director of Program Services of the Alzheimer's Association of Minnesota, "Alzheimer's disease reminds me of cancer twenty years ago. The biggest question was, 'Should we tell the patient?' It's been called the big A. Cancer twenty years ago was called the big C. Our goal is to eliminate fear and develop understanding so that people can be helped with the disease process."

There is some frustration on the part of families and caregivers alike when it comes to impacting the awareness level of the professional community, most particularly doctors and clergymen. It takes a lot of time to work with people with dementia and their families. According to John Kitto, recent Executive Director of the Alzheimer's Association of Minnesota, "Alzheimer's disease represents dilemmas, social dilemmas. For the most part, doctors don't know how to deal with this. Families put doctors on a pedestal, but increasingly doctors have to produce a certain amount of revenue. Talking with the family of an Alzheimer's patient isn't going to get it for them."

Julie Nygren, the former Family Services Director, agrees. She says it's not the doctor you talk to about the practical problems of Alzheimer's disease, it's someone else. She feels that the contact person at the doctor's office or clinic is the best link in the education process. It is the contact person who can share information from the Alzheimer's Association and other sources with patients as well as be a referral source for support groups and other services. Nygren makes the point that the only thing the consumer can't get from a nonphysician is medication.

"Our hope," says Cheryl Biel, "is to get the doctor, nurses, and office staff to say, 'Call the Alzheimer's Association.' If we can get them to come to our door, we can help direct them to services."

Most Alzheimer's associations around the country still grapple with the enormous challenges of serving large geographic areas with light staffing and limited budgets. However, the vision for the future at the Minnesota Lakes office is to continue to develop regional offices in outstate areas and to foster awareness of the Association and its services through Memory Walk fund-raisers, where walkers are sponsored by people in the community who make monetary pledges that fund research and services. The Minnesota walk, now in its tenth year, is the largest Memory Walk in the nation.

The money raised goes to research, to setting up special-care units for Alzheimer's disease patients, and to working with assisted living and foster-care facilities. The Association's commitment is to work as a team with the community and to learn from one another.

"There is no right or wrong answer to this disease," says Bobbie Speich, former Chapter Services Director. "You learn because every day is different. I think that's why medical people get so frustrated. They want the right answer."

John Kitto agrees: "Unless physicians have had someone in their family or a good friend with Alzheimer's disease, they are a hard group to crack. Physicians try to go from point A to point B. They are problem solvers. Their world is medicine, not human services. "

Dr. David Knopman, one of the most available and responsive physicians I have ever worked with, says, "People need a game plan for how to access community services and how to decide on other issues like finances, place of residence, even the appropriateness of driving a car. Physicians in general don't have that expertise, which is arguably outside the medical model. It would be nice, but it may be asking too much." He does say, however, that physicians need resources to which they can refer people.

Aside from working with the few visionaries that exist in the medical arena—such as Dr. Jonathan Evans, his colleague Dr. Eric Tangelos, Dr. David Knopman, and others around the country—John Kitto feels trying to educate the medical community is like hitching your wagon to the wrong star.

He asserts that awareness and change will be driven by consumers and their loved ones. Families that have had a positive experience in a smaller home setting will not remain quiet. They learn first-hand that there are options besides nursing home care, that it is possible to maintain the quality of their loved one's life; they learn about ways to respond to the special needs of Alzheimer's patients. That is what will drive the demand for models that fit and caregivers who respond.

Special Needs of People With Alzheimer's Disease
Educating the caregivers is another area that must be addressed as we look to the future.

In the last seven years the assisted-living phenomenon has blossomed. Assisted-living facilities provide lovely apartments with congregate dining as an option, along with other services such as help with bathing, house cleaning, and exercise provided on a contract basis. Although assisted living is a wonderful, workable alternative for many elderly people, many who work with memory loss are not convinced that people with dementia can be well served in assisted-living situations for several reasons:

- Although services are available that the person with memory loss needs, the memory loss renders the resident unable to coordinate using them.

- Different providers come different days of the week to provide assisted living services. People with memory loss need consistent staffing with a small number of familiar faces.

- There is not a core supervisory staff to help people with memory loss find their room, the dining room, etc. People with dementia need cueing.

- Because people with dementia need their environment to be kept very simple, it is difficult to assimilate them into an assisted-living situation that has many daily variables. One way to address this might be to create special areas for Alzheimer's residents staffed by specially trained caregivers.

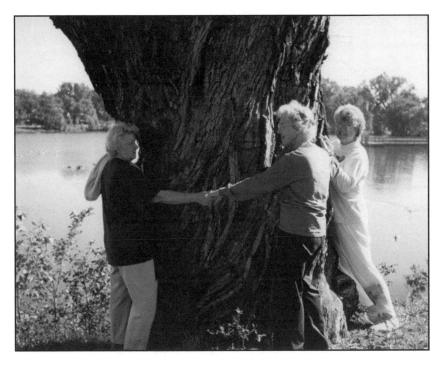

Tree hugging with residents at Lake Como
during Alzheimer's Association Memory Walk

Education of Caregivers

The key thing, according to Dr. Knopman and others, is the personality of
the person working with Alzheimer's disease. Expectations surrounding
communication need to be completely different than with other people. If
those caring for Alzheimer's patients try to communicate as they would
with those who are cognitively intact, the patient will withdraw or get angry.
Successful caregivers are patient and understand limited communication
abilities. They need to know the emotional tone of a verbal exchange even
in absence of actual content. As apparent as this is to our staff and me, as
well as to others who work closely with people with memory loss, many
mainstream caregivers have not had the opportunity to learn how to address
these special needs. Frustration gives way to irritation and everyone loses.

The caregiver has a bad day, and the patient is left with his or her dignity in shreds. (Appendix 2 includes a communication overview.)

The experts who have contributed to this chapter agree with me on this: you can teach caregiving skills and you can impart knowledge about Alzheimer's disease, but if the caregiver doesn't have an open heart, even the best training doesn't make any difference. You have to be careful who you hire, they say; then, with good training, you can overcome other limitations such as less-than-ideal facilities. The Minnesota Lakes Alzheimer's Association developed a train the trainer program called Challenge of Care to help care facilities train their staff members to meet the challenges dementia presents. After all, as Cheryl Biel says, this disease is going to be around for a long time.

One of the key things a model like Rakhma teaches caregivers is that the caregiver must learn from the patient. It's a bit of a dance. Some caregivers have a natural ability to observe and figure things out. Alzheimer's disease does not go by rote. One of the most valuable things to learn is that every day, we don't know. We must pay attention to what is happening right here, right now.

One day I heard a little crackly voice at the Peace Home shouting, "Help, help! Help, help!" I thought one of the residents was stuck somewhere, or had lost her way. I started for the stair to help when I heard the caregiver in charge say, "There, there. Do you want me to hold your hand again, Grace?"

"Yes," croaked the little voice. And all was peaceful again as the helper sat with Grace and held her hand.

What Is Happening to Me? Patient Support Groups

Support groups for families of people with Alzheimer's disease have been around for a long time. They are invaluable tools for bringing about awareness—of the implications of the disease, of one's own feelings, of available resources, and of the beauty of the human spirit. Now the Minnesota Lakes Alzheimer's Association and others around the country sponsor support groups for Alzheimer's patients themselves.

Julie Nygren says they were uncomfortable at first as she and her colleagues grappled with what kinds of things could be dealt with in a group where people were having a hard time remembering.

"We shouldn't have been scared," she reports. "These people are wonderful. If you want to talk about it, they can talk about it. The support groups have been a wonderful learning lab for patients and Alzheimer's Association staff too. Particularly in the early stages, who do the patients have to talk with? The medical community is not making contact with them." The patient support groups help patients and resource people in their efforts to keep life as normal as possible for as long as possible.

Guest speakers who have Alzheimer's disease share stories of how they cope and of what is important to them. In the early stages, says Dr. Knopman, the patient experiences a sense of loss. It can be a frustrating and bewildering time for people, because they know something is wrong, but with their memory loss, they lack the insight to tell what it is.

Sadness or bereavement, he feels, are words that would describe how the family responds to the disease because they have a much greater sense of the future. The disease itself robs the patient of being able to predict the future with much clarity. They are bewildered about what is happening now and not able to see where they will end up.

Support groups give people a sense of community and shared experience, even in their memory loss. It is healing to be able to tell one's story and to listen to the stories of others.

Legislation

In the beginning, I wondered why they couldn't turn nursing homes into the kind of care that we do. Then after being caught up with all the rules that govern houses like ours, I could see how the tangle of rules governing nursing homes can keep them back. Now I'm asking, why couldn't those rules be changed? There are many people in nursing homes who would benefit from a smaller, home-like setting. There have got to be ways that you could change things to make aging a lot friendlier. Maybe it would take buying one of those smaller nursing homes and seeing if you can make some of those changes yourself. Ready. Fire. Aim.

Regulation, though its intention is to safeguard the public, has gotten out of hand. The more regulated the elder-care environment becomes, the less choice the consumer has, and the elderly person often has only one choice—to live in an institutional setting that is based on a medical model. Granted, regulations are necessary. Without them we would have chaos. But perhaps we are operating with outdated paradigms. Certainly it is time to examine how we've always done it.

Kensington Cottages, where Dr. Evans provides medical care, is another innovative model of care for people with memory loss. Says John Rappaport, Executive Director, "The challenge is not to become the regulated model that nursing home care has become. We must make sure policy makers are as educated as possible." What legislators and many of the rest of us don't see, he says, is that safety and security don't give us our quality of life.

After attending a White House Conference on Aging, John put it this way: Mature, middle-aged adults set policy in our society. Their number one concern is that their demented or frail parents don't hurt themselves. They want their loved ones to be safe and secure. They don't see the paradox between what they deem most necessary for others and what they want for themselves. If they were asked, "What do you want?" they would say, "We want the freedom to do what we want to do." If their parents were asked the same thing they would give the same answer, as would their children. However, in making public policy, safety rules. Regulators see themselves as preservers and protectors. The question is, though, how to address the value that our loved ones don't get hurt while keeping in mind the quality of their lives. And quality of life, says John, comes down to relationships with caregivers, the environment people live in, and the opportunity to express what they can express, even if their expression is limited by memory loss or other disabilities.

In a nursing home, safety and security are number one. In a shared home, quality of life is. Laws regulating nursing home safety and security are no longer based on common sense, Rappaport feels, but have gone so far overboard that they take away choice.

States regulate homes under a variety of names, including assisted living facilities, residential care facilities, adult congregate living facilities, personal care homes, catered living facilities, retirement homes, homes for adults, or community residences.

Although legislative bodies make the laws, family members are primary movers in influencing changes in elder-care policy. Family members who have experienced a residential home setting are aware of how it fits the needs of people with memory loss, how the emphasis on quality of life works. Then, informed and spearheaded by the experiences of satisfied family members, a coalition of interested parties, including Alzheimer's disease sufferers, social service organizations, providers, doctors, hospitals, and discharge planners as a group, are in a position help change public policy.

John Kitto of the Alzheimer's Association sees serious challenges for the future. Providing a homelike setting where residents can do things in a natural way is in direct contrast to the currently accepted high-tech systems that emphasize safety and survival at all costs. He feels the small provider must understand the legislative and regulatory realities as well as the powerful realities of money, and with that understanding, work with the rules that are useful and around the ones that aren't.

"Don't have a disaster," he says. "That's what brings on regulatory environments."

He feels it is important to regularly associate with the power brokers in the care industry. He has testified before legislative committees against increasing the regulatory environment for smaller facilities. "There were substantial forces mustered on the other side," he said. "It is essential to make sure that when regulatory issues come up, there is an orchestrated, sophisticated effort to present the point of view of the smaller facility."

John Rappaport has several homes for people with Alzheimer's disease and dementia in outlying areas around Minnesota. His first home was an assisted living facility in a converted hospital building in the town of Buffalo. As an alternative to the local nursing home, it offered services twenty-four hours a day as well a a menu of additional services if they were wanted or needed. Because the nursing home was the only facility for which Medicaid would reimburse and long-term care is expensive, those who started out at John's home ran out of private funds. Forced to go to the nursing home on the other end of town, several former residents had a life they were not happy with, while the taxpayers wound up paying more than if the resident had been able to stay at his Kensington Cottages.

"We went to the state," reported John. "We said we ought to be able to do this. The state's knee-jerk reaction was, 'You are a business man. You just want to make money.' Or the state would say 'Sorry, you're right. It would be cheaper to keep people with you, but federal policy only allows care in certified nursing homes.'"

After advocating "for years and years," John says the regulatory bodies are seeing what a burden care has become and have begun to look at alternatives. In some states, time has brought forth Medicaid waivers, or what are known in Minnesota as Elderly Waivers, which allow people the choice to reside in group residential environments that are not nursing homes. Minnesota is in the forefront of this movement.

These examples, though all from Minnesota, serve to illustrate the kinds of roadblocks that might be or have been encountered in other areas of the nation. According to a 1995 report by the National Academy for State Health Policy, twenty-two states have passed legislation, issued regulations, or started programs through Medicaid home and community-based service programs. Six states have issued draft regulations or have legislation pending. Another five states have created task forces on the issue.

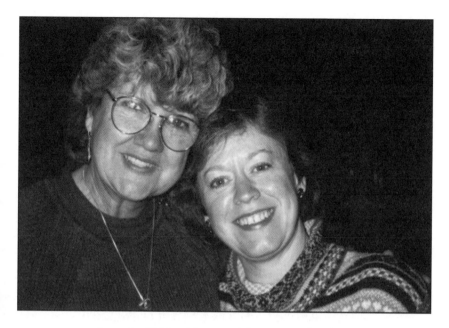

Founder Shirley Shaw and Director Judy Cline

In some states, though, there are also criteria, based on outdated codes that ignore the wishes of the residents and their families, for "appropriate" placement as residents in a personal care home become more frail. This means that people who are simply aging in place and needing more care—maybe they need two people to help transfer them from one place to another, they use a wheelchair, or have dementia—would have to leave their residential home for a nursing home, even though they don't need skilled medical care.

Still another issue is, even in the states where there is funding for residential settings, the uncertain timing of waiver payments impacts cash flow in a smaller setting in a way that it does not in a larger setting where a certain amount of cash-flow fluctuation can be absorbed. This means that smaller settings like Rakhma, though the commitment is to care for everyone regardless of ability to pay, must take a lower percentage of people on Elderly Waiver than they would like or they can't stay afloat.

"We want low-income people to have the option to access this kind of care," says John Rappaport. "I just hope that the Minnesota model, particularly as it affects people with dementia, will not be restricted." If it is, both the resident and the residential home lose.

Staying Alive

Staying in business with alternative housing is fraught with snags. A small residential home pays the same worker's compensation rates as larger nursing homes, even though employees do a variety of jobs and are technically in a different category than workers in a larger facility.

When Rakhma first started, insurers were afraid to cover workers in a small shared home like Rakhma. Covered by Lloyd's of London, Rakhma put out a hunk of money to insure the first home. Next, Rakhma was covered in an insurance pool divied up by different companies. We had and continue to have a very low rate of claims. We were able to get out of the pool for a little while and pay lower premiums until the insurance company that covered us went out of business. Now we're back in the pool. We want to have choices. As it is, we're having to pay monthly because we can't muster the huge insurance premium in one chunk.

Over the past three years Rakhma has been tracking employee caregiving hours separately from employee cleaning/cooking/maintenance hours. Without an internal tracking system, insurers bill premiums based on nursing care only, a much higher rate than for cleaning and maintenance personnel. The differential is six dollars per one hundred dollars in premiums, which translated the first year into a twelve-thousand-dollar savings for Rakhma.

Some of the smaller homes are now being built by larger care centers. This could have happened years ago if the larger centers would have been willing to take less profit. As it is, it's come to the attention of some boards, who have begun to ask, "Why shouldn't we be doing some care in a home setting?" Now a few smaller homes are on large campuses of nursing homes, which can help to absorb the costs of residential care.

However, it's the many, many smaller caregivers I grieve for, and the people whose lives could be enhanced by their care if there were fewer road-blocks to staying in business. One woman in Saint Paul was closing a lovely home as this book was being written. She couldn't make it work financially.

One of John Kitto's key concerns for models like Rakhma is their relationship with the state. "I think it's very important to keep the balance between allowing innovation and allowing greater flexibility without compromising quality," he says. "The problem is that the state and federal governments are under increasing pressure from many factions to increase their surveillance of services offered. The increase in paperwork and increase in inefficiency dictated by generic guidelines puts places like Rakhma at some risk for expansion."

He suggests developing a cost-effective way to document what smaller homes do for both regulatory agencies and consumers so that everything is very clean, easy to see, and specific. Such a self-regulatory system could help more innovative homes avoid the trap of having the state step in and regulate them.

Smaller care facilities have to have twice as many people present to be visible in regulatory meetings. But it is important to have people there. The voices of large nursing homes are loud and adamant. The clear, steady voice of soul-friendly aging must be heard.

The obstacles are enough to dishearten a lot of people. Sometimes I get discouraged too. But we've been here fourteen years now. I feel we have been around long enough to be a voice for change. Even though we operate very close to the line, Rakhma is here to stay. Our homes have provided a model, and that was one of my original intentions.

Consulting

When Rakhma first opened, many people called who wanted to start a home just like it. I have shared my experiences with many people personally, encouraged them, and had follow-up conversations with them on the phone.

There didn't seem to be anyone else doing this when I started, or over the next few years; there were too many roadblocks. During the first few years, I got virtually no calls back reporting openings of new residential homes, but since 1992 more homes have been developed.

Over the years, I began to understand the value of consulting for a fee. I acknowledge that we do have this experience, we've been around a good while now, and it's okay to get paid for our time. And we can choose to give without charge also. In the end, we are accomplishing what we are wanting, to have other homes like ours in other areas.

For the future I see a consulting team, a teaching team, which could help set up homes in other areas and then go on their way after helping hire and train people to staff them.

Modeling for Life

The availability of elder-care models based on lifestyle rather than on medical care offers enormous hope for the future. A new understanding will come as alternative models come into existence. There can't be an effective change of philosophy until there are models for how to do it.

The reality of a residential home model is that the cost is very high. To have enough staff trained to provide care in a quality manner is expensive. The nursing home model was developed around the question of how to give care in the cheapest possible way.

"We know how to do it cheap," says John Rappaport. "That's not possible on a small scale. When you lose one person in a five-person home, you have only eighty-percent occupancy." Perhaps it is time to look at costs other than money. Perhaps making money our prime motivator is part of a crumbling paradigm.

When the business side of caregiving becomes the motivator, it's easy to lose sight of the real purpose for providing care, says Rappaport. "I have evolved to the belief that the nursing home model has become an abysmal failure. Not that there aren't good people, but the system has made it difficult for those people to flourish. Our mission is to help this person who has this horrendous disease to have as good a life as possible for their remaining years."

John's Story—Business with a Commitment

Like so many others who work with Alzheimer's disease, John Rappaport doesn't ask first, "What's in it for me?" He was a real-estate developer who used his business acumen to affect positive change, asking "What's in it for all of us?" He has also had family members with Alzheimer's disease. When asked what called to him about creating shared homes for people with Alzheimer's disease, he told this story:

"When I was a young kid, I was a great student in Hebrew school. There was a time I was asked to recite a prayer in Hebrew: 'And you shall love the Lord your God with all your soul and with all your might, and you shall teach these words unto your children.'

"I was kind of arrogant because I knew the prayer inside out. 'Let other kids fail,' I thought as I watched each one stand up to recite and sit down again because they forgot a word or a line. Then came my moment. The teacher said, 'John, why don't you recite?' I stood up ready to impress everyone with my outstanding grasp of Hebrew, but I couldn't remember the first word. I couldn't remember any of the prayer, so I sat down. The kids laughed. I was so humiliated that I couldn't even read out loud in class after that, although I finally grew out of it.

"My appreciation for memory loss is rooted in that experience. As I look back and think about that time, I see that I had learned the prayer by rote. I had it down cold, but I never, at that age, understood the essence of what the words meant. Forgetting it like I did, though, made me think about it over and over later. The prayer that I had forgotten was all about kindness of heart, the essence of who we are. Even though people may forget words or concepts, they don't forget the kindness of their heart. People don't forget the essence of their being. That incident taught me about the embarrassment of forgetting, and how humiliated people feel when they can't remember and others laugh or become impatient.

"Alzheimer's disease doesn't take away one's essence. It is always there, intact. That is what our work is about."

A Model That Includes Community

Being with each resident, appreciating their essence, and not just treating symptoms of memory loss is what the Rakhma model is based on. It is key to my vision for the future. Without this piece, the rest is just an empty exercise. We in the alternative housing field have the opportunity to look and to say how we are doing our work. We look always at that commitment to love.

When I started Rakhma, I thought that if my staff and I put energy into the houses and got the programs and policies up to snuff, I could eventually put my energy somewhere else. Instead, running a small home is like raising a family. Everything is always ahead of you. There are always going to be things to do in the homes, expenses are always going to go up, regulations are going to change. Policies continually need upgrading. There is no such thing as saying, "This year we're going to get our act together." There will always be the unexpected. It's just the way of life.

If love is the foundation of shared-home care, creativity is the cornerstone. Always there are challenges, maybe more so in the future. I look at the very real possibility that there may not be funding assistance in the future for homes like ours. Does that mean they can't exist?

I put forth the call to community. There are many existing houses in urban and rural areas that may only hold five people that could be made into a Rakhma-style home. The community could provide some supplies and volunteers that, with careful planning, would allow a residential home for the elderly to survive. Somehow, I feel that a small home with only five people, with a good dedicated manager and with community involvement, could be like starting a fire. People could copy the model in their own communities. Maybe there is a house with five in this town, but twenty miles away, in another town, there is another, similar home. Then, in ten or twenty years, there are more, until people see that it is possible to live out one's life affordably and with dignity.

If we really put forth an effort, people can have this option and have much more fun. Many people who don't need medical care could live in a place that is home to them among family, friends, and community.

Shared Homes in Rural Areas

The Rakhma model has been successful in urban areas. There is a great need for good housing in rural areas as well. The plan for such homes would be set up so that a year before a home opens, people in the community would be invited to participate in the project and in doing so begin to feel some ownership. The plan would seek volunteer commitments from churches, civic organizations, and retired people for meals and things such as rides to doctors.

I would look for a farmhouse or a large house in town that could be remodeled, possibly something that Habitat for Humanity would help with, or church members or the Rotary or the Elks. It could even be that an organization of committed people would own the home and Rakhma would train the managers and consult on a long term-basis as needed.

They say, "How could you afford to do this when there are only six hundred people in the whole town?" There are people from all around the towns, too. I've been told something like this would be well received. Even within a fifty-mile radius, families are willing to drive that distance for this choice.

A place on a lake would be ideal. Or another possibility would be an old hotel, near a community pool where we could take our residents to swim or watch the kids swimming. Maybe there would be a senior center up the way, a little beauty shop and a grocery store. The possibilities are endless.

People talk: "How can you expect to find volunteers in rural areas when you can't easily find them in the cities?" In my optimism I think, if we find the home, they will come! In outlying areas there are many hard-working farm folks. I visualize soups cooking, bread baking, people coming in to read and to have fun. I believe providing transportation for our volunteers would help bring them in. My desire is to have a model that doesn't have to start off with private pay for a year and a half.

Among retired folk, I am seeing that there is such a huge group of people who could be so much more involved. Along with Rakhma's involvement in alternative housing for the elderly, we can also be a connecting, networking voice with those who care about how the elderly are treated, in utilizing our resources, using people whose lives might otherwise become narrow. Our need as human beings is to be connected with and needed by others. If we're no longer needed in that CEO position or that sales position or no longer raising children, it doesn't mean we can't still put forth that energy to work on something that matters. I love to get involved in a project. Don't we all need something to look forward to? We can start right in our own community

Finances

We definitely need some support for our programs. We have to reframe with new tactics and a new plan. A professional development person volunteered his services to Rakhma. He went on to become a board member and is training management and board members in the ways of fund-raising, proposal writing, and networking. Foundations may be one avenue and private donors another. New board members are being recruited who have a commitment to quality care as well as financial connections in the community. A volunteer committee called the Rakhma Angels makes phone calls and sets up visits and presentations with neighborhood churches, building relationships and letting church staff know about Rakhma as a resource for members who may need elder care now or in the future. More and more partnership is being developed with individuals, organizations, and the community at large.

Partnership

In the caregiving field there has been a great split coming out of the old paradigm of competition. Rifts abound between groups around the country—home-like care versus corporate care, profit versus nonprofit. That's not reality, suggests the staff at the Minnesota Lakes Alzheimer's Association. Instead of working against each other, let's work together. Looking at it another way would suggest that with many models there is something for everyone.

The Buddhists say there are three mysteries: water to the fish, air to the bird, and the human being to himself or herself. It is only when the fish is taken out of water that the fish knows water. Otherwise water is experienced as indistinct from fish. The bird only knows air, distinct from itself, when taken out of air. We have a Self that is separate and distinct, but we don't know Self until we step aside from the backdrop "human being." Only then do we have the freedom to use our human being-ness consciously to create something other than what has always been. We step out of the water we swim in to see it clearly for the first time. We ask the question of ourselves, "If I am Self, separate from all my circumstances, reactions, thoughts, feelings, and opinions, then what is this Self up to?" This is the opening for a future that is by conscious design, not more of the same with variations.

Partnership is a concept that's been around a long time, one we think we are familiar with, but perhaps not so. The water we swim in as human beings in this culture is that of win/lose. Competition dominates the business world and the health-care field; it is air we breathe.

To live in partnership, to *live* partnership, requires making a complete shift. We don't know how to be partners, for partnership means facing the unknown. Who do we have to be to be partners, to mentor one another, to think in terms of "we," not "us/them"? Who do we have to be to do business with integrity, to look at not only the financial costs but to include the costs in human suffering and the benefits of human dignity into decision-making equations? Who do we have to be to respond to one another as human beings in the business world, as caregivers and in our personal lives? Who do we have to be to live as partners each day of our lives?

What we do comes out of who we are being. As partners we educate. We include community. We empower volunteers. We open our hearts. We learn from our dear friends and loved ones with Alzheimer's disease.

Partnership is where we go from here if the quality of life for older people, and all people on the planet, is to be cultivated lovingly, like a great, beautiful garden.

To Keep in Mind...

- Love is the foundation and creativity is the cornerstone of shared-home care, now and in the future.

- Shared homes introduce a quality-of-life model of care for the future that provides a viable option for people who do not need or desire a medical-model setting.

- Shared homes pioneer the viability of business with commitment.

- Shared homes bring back the concept of the honored elder.

- Education—in the classroom, in the professions, of caregivers—must affect us personally. We can then make an impact in our homes and families, as well in the larger community.

- Legislative changes will be grass-roots driven. As more and more people experience the benefits of shared-home care, their voices will make the difference.

- Community involvement in elder care will include resource groups like the national and regional Alzheimer's associations, physicians, clergy, family and friends of the elderly, as well as volunteer organizations, churches, and schools.

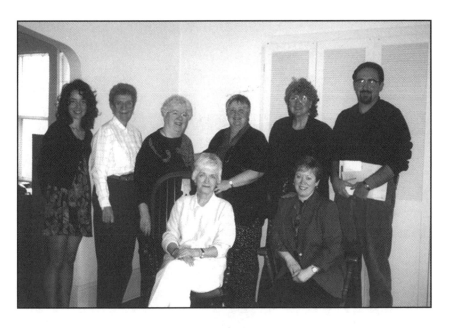

Board of Directors
Back row: Michelle Jenson (staff), Barb Norling, Mary Ondov, Trish Herbert, Shirley Shaw, and Colin MacKenzie; front row: Carol Fredrickson and Judy Cline

- Consulting services are available at Rakhma to help support and develop shared homes around the country.

- The use of existing housing in cities and rural areas makes good use of resources, provides a homelike atmosphere, and builds community.

- Developing partnerships within the elder-care community makes a win/win future possible.

- Shared homes are here to stay.

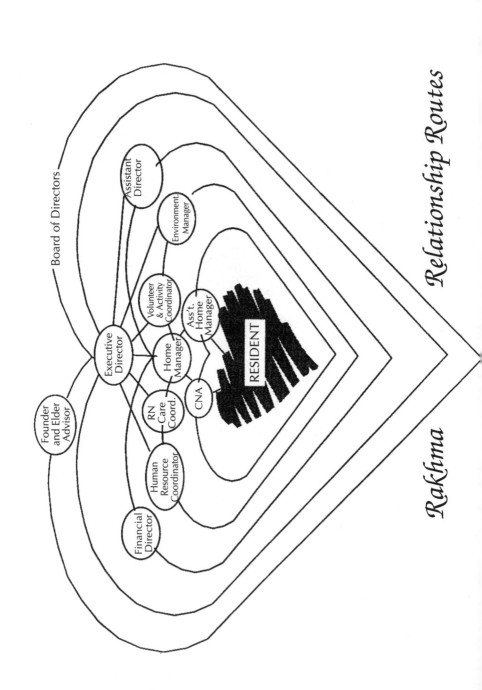

Rakhma   Relationship Routes

Appendix I

The Rakhma Model

Philosophy

The name *Rakhma* (Rok'-ma) is an ancient Aramaic word meaning unconditional love. Rakhma, Inc., is committed to providing loving care to the elderly residents of our shared community homes. We are dedicated to preserving their dignity and encouraging the natural expression of joy in their lives. Based on a philosophy of creativity, harmony, and love, Rakhma is willing to go the extra mile to provide service with a heart.

Heart Chart—Rakhma Organizational Chart

Shown on facing page. Brief job descriptions follow:

Team Staff

Team Mission—The Rakhma Team consists of management and administrative staff whose purpose is to direct, assist, and support the managing staff in individual Rakhma homes, with a goal of fostering the philosophy of unconditional love and service with a heart at all levels of our organization. While there are clearly supervisory relationships between certain of these team members and staff members in our houses, the primary desire of the Team is to provide the resources and tools needed by the homes to make the Rakhma philosophy a reality. It is also the mission of the Team to live out the philosophy in our relationships with each other and all the Rakhma staff members.

Executive Director—Oversees all Rakhma operations to see that philosophy of care is carried out in all areas. Duties include community outreach;

supervising personnel and making personnel policies; and creating financial, licensing, insurance, and safety structures with input from consultants
and the Board of Directors.

Founder-Elder Advisor Consultant—Shirley Joy Shaw's personal job description—at age 63: consulting, problem-solving, providing leadership and service wherever needed.

RN Care Coordinator—Through weekly on-site visits with the residents, the
RN assures that the health and safety needs of all residents are met. The RN
sees to it that staff training in medical policies and procedures are current
through reviews and staff in-services. The RN also consults with doctors and
families of the residents, acts as a resource to staff regarding medical issues,
and assists in maintaining compliance with current regulations and standards.
    Specific duties include assisting in assessment of new residents, care
planning and discharge decisions as well as providing ongoing nursing support and consultation by phone and regularly scheduled visits to each home.

Human Resource Coordinator—Coordinates personnel, training, benefits,
and affirmative action and acts as a general administrative assistant. Also
attends conferences and exhibits to foster good community relations.

Assistant Director—Provides management support. Directs admissions,
marketing, and advertising. Specific duties include working with families
through the intake and admission process, serving as a referral and education source for families and area agencies, representing the Rakhma model
through exhibits at local conferences, producing the *Rakhma Heartbeat*
newsletter twice a year, and managing an annual promotional budget.

Activity Coordinator—Coordinates special events, daily activities, in-house
events, and weekly activities. Duties include coordinating the Rakhma van

outings and maintaining the van, encouraging the talents of staff members, interacting with residents' families, gathering material and nonmaterial resources, and community networking and education.

Volunteer Coordinator—Develops and coordinates the volunteer program in all homes. Coordinates residents' needs with volunteer talent. Specific duties include helping assess each resident's leisure needs; recruiting, interviewing, and training volunteers; coordinating volunteer opportunities with each house; and community networking and education.

Financial Director—Oversees all financial aspects of Rakhma, including financial statements, budgeting, annual certified audit, payroll, accounts receivable and third party billing, accounts payable, banking, applicable taxes, and insurance. Advises Co-directors and Board of Directors to achieve the most effective use of resources.

Environmental Manager—Maintains and improves the Rakhma property and grounds, performs scheduled maintenance and emergency repairs, inventories property and inventories, and purchases bulk supplies and food.

Support Staff

Home Manager—Responsible for quality of care of the residents and creating a smoothly run home under the Rakhma concept of care. Supervises all activities of employees within the home.

Care duties include supervising care of residents, ordering medications, and coordinating medication sheets under RN supervision. Communicates with residents' families regarding personal funds, personal supply needs, concerns about resident. Sometimes works on the floor as a certified nursing assistant (CNA), fulfilling the CNA job description.

Household duties include ordering and purchasing operating supplies, planning menus, supervising grocery shopping, and overseeing cleanliness of the premises.

Staffing and educational duties include assisting in interview process, supervising orientation and training, coaching staff, scheduling and holding monthly staff meetings.

Assistant Home Manager—Provides direct quality care to residents and assists the Home Manager in maintaining a smoothly running home under the Rakhma concept of care. Helps supervise all activities of employees within the home. Fills in for the Home Manager as necessary.

Specific duties include working on the floor as a CNA, fulfilling the CNA job description, as well as assisting the Home Manager in most areas (see Home Manager).

Certified Nursing Assistant (CNA)—Provides direct quality care to residents living at Rakhma.

Specific duties include giving complete personal care; administering medication (after taking a medication administration course); spending time with residents one-on-one; involving residents in activities such as music, games, walks, reading, etc.; housekeeping; cooking; welcoming visitors; and attending staff meetings and in-services. He or she also completes all required documentation such as verbal reports; entries in the communication, medication, staff meeting, and in-service logs; and filing incident reports.

Elements of the Rakhma Model

- Quality of life emphasis; non-medical model
- Use of existing housing in existing neighborhoods and communities
- Staff ratio one to four or one to five; shift staffing

- Overall structure that makes day-to-day flexibility and appropriate response to residents possible

- Family involvement

- Creation of family atmosphere with residents and staff in the shared-home setting

- Activities that involve residents in living as normal a life as possible

- Provision for aging in place

- Provision for dying in the home

- Continuum of care for those who move to other settings

- Participation of volunteers

- A vision for the future that includes making the Rakhma model available to communities around the nation, education for families, schools and churches, legislative support of alternative care models, and partnership with other care providers to ensure a full spectrum of choices for those who need care.

Appendix 2

Educational Curriculum Suggestions

Schools

Objective: To foster understanding of older people among elementary school children.

Means: A retired volunteer spends one hour a week for five weeks in a third- through fifth-grade classroom using the following guidelines for lesson plans.

Week 1: Exploration

Introductions.

Who do you know that is old?

What does it mean to get old?

Older person tells a story about his or her grandmother or grandfather.

Any stories about your grandparents?

Anyone in the neighborhood who is old? Could you meet them this week, say hi?

Notice how old people are portrayed on television this week. In the movies you watch.

Week 2: Playtime

Check in: Did talk to anyone who is older this week? What did you ask them?

What did you notice about older people from the TV or movies you watched?

What kinds of things do you like to do for fun?

The volunteer tells about something he or she liked to do for fun.

Share a song or a poem from when the volunteer was a child.

Play a game with the group that the older person played when a child.

Homework: Ask a grandparent or neighbor about games they liked to play when they were children. Have them teach one to you.

Week 3: School

Check in: Who did something with an older person last week? What did you do? What did you learn?

Have kids tell what their school day is like. How do they get there? How far do they go? What are their subjects? What is available to help learn (computers, media center, etc.)? What is their favorite subject, their toughest?

Volunteer tells story of a typical day at school. What were his or her biggest concerns? How were the children disciplined? Did they have field trips? What was recess like? Tell about a big success in school, or an embarrassing moment in school.

Homework: Have kids ask grandparents, older neighbor about school.

Week 4: The process of aging

Check in: Share about conversations with older people about school or anything else.

Conversation about noticing older people in their neighborhood, at church, in the store, etc.

Talk about changes that older people experience. Talk about grandpa, grandma, aunt, uncle, who may do or say some funny things sometimes. Then talk about memory-loss disease, what it is.

(Brief overview in packet for volunteer to work from.)

Talk about changes in volunteer's life, physically, mentally, emotionally.

Talk about concerns older people have.

Homework: Have children ask older person about changes, good and bad, that they experience with age.

<u>Week 5: Bringing it together</u>

Draw a picture of a favorite memory of a time you spent with an older person. Or, if they have no older people in their life, draw a picture of what you and an older person could do together. Share about these pictures.

Who are the older people in your life? Have you made any new older friends? Have you gotten to know anyone better? What memories have you made since we began? What can you do to create more good memories with the older people in your life? How can you encourage your parents to include older people more?

Community Presentation / Lecture

<u>Outline</u>

Alzheimer's Association and residential home partnership (two speakers per event) or, one speaker from residential home presenting to church groups, community organizations, civic organizations, etc.

I. Aging and dementia overview
   A. It's not just a part of "getting old"
   B. Statistics (source: Alzheimer's Association)
II. Warning signs and symptoms
   A. More than forgetful (when to be concerned)
   B. Medical evaluation—ruling out other causes
   C. Diagnosis
III. Coping
   A. Changing behaviors
   B. Family stresses
   C. Changing the environment
   D. Support resources (Alzheimer's Association, doctor, family, support groups, etc.)
IV. When to seek help
   A. Vulnerability

    B. Safety issues

    C. Caregiver survival

 V. What are the options?

    A. Home care

    B. Day care

    C. Alternative living arrangements, including:

       1. Assisted living

       2. Nursing homes

       3. Creative community options

In-service for Care Facilities

<u>Overview</u>

Participants might include: hospitals, nursing homes, group homes; nurses, social workers, caregivers, volunteers.

In addition to Alzheimer's disease, other conditions can cause memory loss: cancer, AIDS, Parkinson's disease, etc. Even people who are mentally disabled often experience memory loss as they move into their forties.

The following is an outline of an in-service training that covers how to work with people who have memory loss in respectful and life-enhancing ways:

  I. Why difficult behaviors occur

    A. Causes related to the person's physical and emotional health

      • Effects of medications.

      • Impaired vision or hearing.

      • Acute illness, chronic illness, physical discomfort.

      • Dehydration, constipation.

      • Depression, fatigue.

    B. Causes related to the environment

      • Environment is too large.

      • There is too much clutter.

- There is excessive stimulation.
- There is no orientation information (cues).
- The environment has poor lighting and/or visual contrasts.
- The environment is unstructured (no routine).

C. Causes related to the task

- Task is too complicated.
- There are too many steps combined.
- Task has not been modified for increasing impairments.
- Task is unfamiliar.

II. What not to do when communicating with a resident

A. Don't argue.

B. Don't order resident around.

C. Don't tell the resident what he or she can't do.

D. Don't be condescending.

E. Don't ask a lot of direct questions that rely on good memory.

F. Don't talk about resident when he or she is in the room.

III. Why dementia residents need special communication

A. Brain damage

B. To validate

C. Inability to interpret environment like people without memory loss

D. To reduce failure in everyday life

E. To distract and redirect behavior

In-services are interactive. They include sharing experiences caregivers have had with residents who exhibit difficult behavior, sharing thoughts on why residents benefit from special communication, and role playing the use of communication skills to de-escalate agitated behavior.

APPENDIX 3

Resources

Rakhma, Inc.
4953 Aldrich Avenue South
Minneapolis, Minnesota 55419
(612) 824–2345
Fax: (612) 824-3165
Consulting and speaking on unconditional love and caring for people with
Alzheimer's disease, dementia, memory loss, and related disorders.

National Alzheimer's and Related Disorders Association
919 North Michigan Avenue
Suite 1000
Chicago, Illinois 60611–1676
Information and referral line: (800) 272–3900
Fax: (312) 335-1110
Web site: www.alz.org/

- Alzheimer's disease information
- Caregiver classes
- Community resources
- Speakers' bureau
- Regional referral
- Books and videotapes
- Caregiving information
- Professional training
- Support groups

The Reagan Research Institute

Part of the National Alzheimer's Association. Builds cooperative relationships among scientists, pharmaceutical and biotech companies, universities and medical centers, private foundations and government. Also puts together collaborative "drug discovery teams" to find effective new treatments for Alzheimer's disease.

For more information call (800) 272-3900.

Alzheimer's Association
Minnesota Lakes Chapter
4570 West 77th Street
Suite 198
Edina, Minnesota 55435
(800) 830-0512
Fax: (612) 830-0513

This is is just one regional chapter that will provide you with facts about Alzheimer's disease, a broad spectrum of information and services for caregivers, patient services information, and alternative housing resources. Call the National Alzheimer's Disease Association (noted earlier) to find your closest chapter.

National Directory of Alzheimer's Specific Residential Care Programs,
    1996
Foxwood Springs Living Center
Foxwood Springs Institute
1500 W. Foxwood Drive
P.O. Box 1172
Raymore, Missouri 64083
(816) 331-3311

Information on specialized Alzheimer's programs in residential settings throughout the United States. Four hundred providers listed.

Alzheimer's Care Consultants
1500 W. Foxwood Drive
P.O. Box 1172
Raymore, Missouri 64083
(816) 331-331, ext. 237
Assistance with the development of:
  • Assisted living specialized Alzheimer's programs
  • Skilled nursing Alzheimer's special care units
  • Specialized Alzheimer's staff education and training

Assisted Living Today
10300 Eaton Place
Suite 400
Fairfax, Virginia 22030
A comprehensive, lively magazine published by the Assisted Living Facilities Association of America; includes stories on issues from policy making to financing to legal concerns faced by facilities and residents of this care option. Always, the dignity of the resident, the heart of what a nonmedical model is about, shines through.
1 year, $16.

Alzheimer's Disease Education & Referral Center (ADEAR)
P.O. Box 8250
Silver Springs, Maryland 20907-8250
Phone: (800) 438-4380
Fax: (301) 587-4352
Web site: www.alzheimers.org.adear
A service of the National Institute on Aging. The Center provides health professionals, patients and their families, and the general public information about Alzheimer's disease diagnosis, treatment, resources, and research. Its resources include brochures, booklets, fact sheets, bibliographies, training programs, congressional reports, and referrals.

Minnesota Health & Housing Alliance
2550 University Avenue West
Suite 3305
Saint Paul, Minnesota 55114–1900
Phone: (651) 645-4545
Fax: (651) 645-0002
Toll Free: (800) 462–5368
A statewide trade association consisting of providers if a complete continuum of services for older adults, including nursing home care, senior housing with supportive services, and community-based services. It is one of
the largest trade associations of its type in the country, and is nationally
recognized for its leadership on long-term care and related issues. MHHA
counts among its members nearly 250 nonprofit nursing homes and more
than 270 senior housing communities, plus all the related services offered
by their organizations. The Minnesota Health & Housing Alliance name
reflects the rapid changes which are taking place in older adult services.
MHHA's members are dedicated to helping people live as independently
as possible through the provision of health care, housing, and community-
based services.

Metropolitan Area Agency on Aging, Inc.
1600 University Ave. W.
Suite 300
Saint Paul, Minnesota 55104–3825
Phone: (651) 641-8612
Fax: (651) 641-8618
Senior Linkage Line: (800) 333–2433
Web site: www.teaging.org.
The purpose of the Area Agency on Aging is to help elders to age suc-
cessfully. For more than twenty-five years, the Metropolitan Area Agency
on Aging has helped elderly throughout the Minneapolis-Saint Paul area

enhance their ability to contribute to society as they grow older and to remain independent by creating and sustaining a system of nutrition and supportive services. The agency is a focal point for:

- Planning and coordinating the efforts of many aging supportive service providers
- Concerns regarding the elderly
- Ensuring ease of access to services
- Leveraging Older Americans Act funds for maximum benefit
- Linking people with information
- Making communities good places to grow old

To order additional copies of this book,
please send full amount plus $4.00 for
postage and handling for the first book and
50¢ for each additional book.

Send orders to:

Galde Press, Inc.
PO Box 460
Lakeville, Minnesota 55044-0460

Credit card orders call 1–800–777–3454
Phone (612) 891–5991 • Fax (612) 891–6091
Visit our website at http://www.galdepress.com

Write for our free catalog.